TREATING THE SELF

TREATING THE SELF

Elements of Clinical Self Psychology

ERNEST S. WOLF, M.D.

The Guilford Press
New York London

© 1988 The Guilford Press
A Division of Guilford Publications, Inc.
72 Spring Street, New York, NY 10012

Printed in the United States of America

Last digit is print number: 9 8 7 6 5 4 3 2

Library of Congress Cataloging in Publication Data

Wolf, Ernest S.
  Treating the self / Ernest S. Wolf.
    p. cm.
  Bibliography: p.
  Includes index.
  ISBN 0-89862-717-6
  1. Self. 2. Psychoanalysis. I. Title.
  [DNLM: 1. Ego. 2. Psychoanalysis. 3. Psychoanalytic Therapy.
4. Self Assessment (Psychology) WM 460.5.E3 W853e]
RC489.S43W65   1988
616.89'17—dc19
DNLM/DLC
for Library of Congress   88-4860
                                                          CIP

TO INA

PREFACE

This book is about how an analyst analyzes, from the point of view of psychoanalytic self psychology. Psychoanalysts are blessed with a plentiful literature, and one may well ask what justifies adding one more book to the plethora of current and valued past publications. In my judgment there is a gap in this massive psychoanalytic literature. What is needed is a text that will bridge the hiatus between, on the one hand, the abundant theoretical discussions in the psychoanalytic corpus and, on the other hand, the extensive published case histories and vignettes that have been chosen to illustrate various points of view with clinical findings. In this volume I have tried to avoid elaborating theory and have accepted the main body of psychoanalytic self psychology as put forth by Kohut and his colleagues during the last two decades. My main focus has been on the application of the self-psychological conception of the psyche to the conduct of psychoanalytic treatment. However, that does not mean a "how-to" book on psychoanalytic practice, but an extraction of guidelines for thinking about therapy, perhaps implying a theory of treatment.

In order to convey the usefulness of the psychoanalytic approach described in this book, this account would have to evoke in the reader the psychoanalytic experience of both analyst and analysand. Within the limitations of the written word, I have striven to accomplish this goal. Psychoanalysis is best carried on in a spirit of open inquiry that is not constrained even by the bounds of theory. Ideally, the analyst keeps his mind hovering evenly and the analysand keeps associating freely, goals that one can aim for but that are equally difficult, if not impossible, to reach perfectly. Therefore, I do not believe that it is very helpful in conducting an analytic treatment to fashion a detailed treatment plan based on extensive diagnostic investigations before beginning the analysis. Rather, in practice, it is best to let diagnosis and treatment evolve in an interactive process with the analysand. Still, for heuristic purposes, I cannot avoid a certain amount of classifying and systematizing, especially as a book has to be written in chapters that group together topics and ideas. Treatment, however, is not carried out that way. At best, after an analysis has terminated, one can, in retrospect, organize a systematic description of what occurred. Such descriptions then can become useful for communicating with others about the issues of psychoanalytic theory and practice.

Inevitably, writing about how an analyst analyzes is a very personal statement. Doing psychoanalysis is an endeavor that is soaked through with the subtle participation of both analyst and analysand. A fruitful discussion that is clinically relevant cannot, therefore, avoid altogether expressing the personality as well as the scientific views of the analyst. As already mentioned, the psychoanalytic theory that has informed and guided my thinking in this book is the body of knowledge that has come to be known as the psychoanalytic psychology of the self. Self psychology is the corpus of the work of Heinz Kohut as he formulated it and as it is being elaborated, modified, and developed by his colleagues and students. In writing this book, I have liberally quoted, paraphrased, and otherwise borrowed not only from Heinz Kohut and his colleagues, but also from my previous publications. Whenever it seemed appropriate, I have given references to the publications of Kohut and his colleagues, but undoubtedly there have been inadvertent but important omissions for which I apologize.

In spite of the sometimes somewhat shrill debates that have accompanied the discussion of self psychology among psychoanalysts, the controversies raging around its major ideas seem to be slowly waning. Kohut's ideas are gradually modifying the theories and practice of most psychoanalysts and other psychotherapists. There is an understandable reluctance on the part of tradition-minded psychoanalysts to use Kohut's terminology, so that some of his ideas surface in ostensibly more classical psychoanalytic expositions under cover of the classical terms that have been subtly redefined to take on aspects of their Kohutian meanings. In view of the gradual absorption of self-psychological thinking into the mainstream of psychoanalysis, I sometimes find it advisable to contrast Kohut's ideas with more traditional ways of doing psychoanalytic treatment. There are two reasons for this. First, from a heuristic point of view, contrasting often dramatically highlights differences that are important but otherwise might remain unnoticed. Second, I want to make sure that Kohut's name be associated with the modifi-

cations that he originated. (Heinz Kohut died in 1981. The reader
may gain some glimpses into his life and his work from Strozier,
1985; Miller, 1985; and Meyers, 1988.) My record in having published contributions to the history of psychoanalysis and biographical
studies of Sigmund Freud testify to the undiminished respect I have
for the genius who founded our science. Nevertheless, it is my
conviction that the mainstream of the psychoanalysis of the future
will be very much like, if not identical with, what we call self
psychology today—until the day arrives that some even newer and
more encompassing set of ideas will be found to advance the psychoanalytic enterprise.

Ernest Wolf

CONTENTS

TREATING THE SELF

.I.

THE PSYCHOLOGY OF THE SELF

. 1 .

INTRODUCTION: HISTORICAL DEVELOPMENT

Psychoanalysis was the creation of Sigmund Freud. Formulated during the waning days of the nineteenth century and elaborated during the initial four decades of the twentieth, Freud's thinking first originated and then dominated the theories and the practice of psychoanalysis and its applications. The novel idea of the mind as being not only coextensive with consciousness, but including also a vast unconscious has remained the *sine qua non* of any psychological theorizing that aims to be psychoanalytic. Indeed, the extent to which the concept of the unconscious mind has become an accepted and integral, if tacitly assumed, part of popular culture in Western society is a measure of the penetration and permanent revolution set in motion by Freud's ideas.

In common with all pioneering scientists, Freud's achievements rest on the shoulders of his predecessors. He did not invent the idea of unconscious experience, nor was he the first to recognize it. Freud probably would have acknowledged that the credit for this discovery should go to the poets, especially Cervantes, Shakespeare, and Goethe, at whose feet Freud became a psychologist. (cf. Gedo & Pollock, 1976, pp. 71–111) Similarly, other fundamental Freudian ideas were as much a product of his immersion into tragedy and novel as they were the result of the systematic study of his patients, and, especially, of himself. Had one asked him the origin of the concept of the oedipus complex, he might well have answered, as the name implies, Sophocles or perhaps Shakespeare's Hamlet (cf. Jones, 1954). Freud's achievement was to take seriously the unconscious forces that he believed had shaped the Western cultural tradition. He studied them systematically and built them into that great and sprawlingly untidy theoretical structure called psychoanalysis.

Psychoanalysis, however, is more than a system of concepts and more than an instrument for research into unconscious motivations and experience. It is also a method for the psychological treatment of certain psychological disorders. Often it is thought that psychoanalysis developed out of hypnosis—especially the hypnotherapeutic attempts of the French neurologists Bernheim, Janet, and Charcot, with whom Freud studied (Ellenberger, 1970; Miller *et al.*, 1969). However, the origins of the clinical method that is peculiarly psychoanalytic are actually to be found in Breuer's management of his famous patient Anna O. Breuer was at this time still using hypnosis to elicit repressed memories (Pollock, 1968)—as Freud did later, initially. However, Breuer had already initiated the fundamental innovation of substituting prolonged empathic immersion for the hypnotic process as the preferred method of data collection par excellence in what later came to be called psychoanalysis. Freud amply credited Breuer for basic clinical psychoanalytic discoveries. Breuer was gifted and renowned as both scientist and researcher. He discovered and described basic neurophysiological phenomena, for example, in his studies of the vestibular system and of the respiratory system's Hering-Breuer reflex which carries his name. Though Breuer was, like Freud, one of the leading medical investigators of his time, he also was a busy practitioner with a wide and varied practice. It is in this latter capacity that Breuer made his most important contribution to clinical psychoanalysis. In retrospect it seems astonishing that such a busy physician found the time and energy to visit Anna O. day after day, week after week, to patiently listen to her symptoms and her story, hour after hour, observing and recording all the while. This was not the usual way that physicians treated hysterical patients. On the other hand, Anna O. was a unique person in her own right. Some years later, Breuer reported his unprecedented encounter with her to Freud. Freud transformed Breuer's apparently singular experience into a systematic method for the exploration and medical treatment of the psyche. Thus psychoanalysis was born when Freud's philosophical–theoretical formulations were fertilized by Breuer's clinical findings and then subjected by Freud to systematic study. This interplay between theory and clinic still characterizes psychoanalysis today.

Psychoanalysis thus is not just a theory, but also a method for probing into the depths of the human psyche. Furthermore, this method has a therapeutic potential. Freud did not enjoy being a physician. For a long time he felt a greater kinship to his idealized mentors in the basic physiological and neuroanatomical sciences, and he became a noted laboratory researcher. His decision to enter medical practice was made reluctantly in response to the pressing need to support a wife and growing family. Even so, he remained in attitude a researcher and disclaimed any great therapeutic ambitions. Confronted in the practice of neurology with the puzzling conditions that today we call the neuroses, Freud developed out of Breuer's experience with Anna O. a method for the treatment of hysteria, which he later extended to the other neuroses. Bringing together the analysis of symptoms, of dreams, and of parapraxes, such as slips of the tongue, he proposed a basic model for the structure of psychoneurotic phenomena. In essence, he saw the neurotic symptom as a compromise structure, which he held to consist of an infantile sexual drive that has leaped across the repression barrier—thus threatening the ego—and been contained by defensive modification and neutralization.

Let me illustrate with an example that is a condensed and simplified but didactically useful version of a case, a boy, whom I treated many years ago.

A naturally curious youngster will be intensely interested in the mysteries of sex and where babies come from. In a bourgeois family of fin de siècle Vienna such matters were not to be talked about directly and openly, especially with children. The boy's curiosity, however, got the better of him and when he was caught spying on his sister in the bath he was reprimanded severely. Some years later, as a young adult, he suddenly became blind, but no organic–biological basis for his blindness was found. A diagnosis of hysterical blindness was confirmed when his sight returned during the course of psychological treatment. It became evident that the blindness had occurred in the context of a sexually tempting situation where he feared his unacceptable sexual interest would be observed. According to the classical psychoanalytic model of symptom formation, we would postulate that his voyeurism of early childhood represented infantile sexual wishes emerging from his id; these had to be repressed into the unconscious because the scolding he received for his boldness became associated with fantasies of a perceived threat of castration. When, as a young adult, a sexually stimulating situation provoked a renewed activity of the repressed impulses, the latter intruded into his ego, where the associated threat of castration now evoked protective measures, the defenses. At the behest of his conscience—

his superego—the ego activated a defensive reaction of an inability to see, that is, the blindness. Yet, the compromise structure of the symptoms is evident in that he can now satisfy his impulse to look, albeit without seeing.

Psychoanalysis scored many successes in the treatment of such relatively simple symptom neuroses with the method of making the unconscious conscious via interpretation. But the hope of curing all kinds of emotional and mental disturbances was soon disappointed. Patients increasingly sought help with more complicated character and behavior disorders where treatment was difficult and the outcome often unsatisfactory. Many refinements in theory and technique were introduced. Still, a large group of so-called narcissistic and borderline conditions were generally believed to be unanalyzable by American analysts (under the influence of object-relations theories, their British colleagues were more optimistic), even though some modified forms of psychotherapy were deemed helpful.

The development of the concept of the self by Kohut during the '60s and '70s has made contemporary psychoanalysis a much more powerfully therapeutic instrument. At the same time, contemporary psychoanalytic theory, particularly the theories of the psychology of the self, more closely articulate with other contemporary and contiguous sciences of man than do the early classical theories. For instance, the conceptualizations of developmental psychology as they are crystallizing out of observations of infants and mothers seem to fit well with the theories of self psychology (Beebe & Lachmann, 1988; Demos, 1988; Lichtenberg, 1983; Stern, 1985; M. Tolpin, 1986).

A comprehensive study of the evolution of self psychology is an important task for the future. For now it will suffice to put the emergence of the concept of "self" into context: During the early years of psychoanalysis Freud did not clearly distinguish between the colloquial meaning of self and the scientific concept ego. The German term *das Ich* (the I) at that time could refer to either. When Freud first postulated the concept of narcissism, he did not yet view the ego as a structured system within the mind, but used the term *das Ich* to refer to something like the "self" or the "whole person." Narcissism (Freud, 1914) was defined as a stage in psychological development when the child's libido (sexual energies) is invested in (cathects) its own self (*das Ich*). In the early 1920s, with the introduction of the structural point of view, which defines the mental apparatus as the three structures ego, id, and superego, *das Ich* no longer referred to the self, but became the structured system ego.

In an attempt to integrate new insights into a refinement of this structural model of psychoanalysis, Hartmann (1950) undertook to redefine narcissism as the libidinal cathexis of the self rather than of the system ego. The self, according to Hartmann, is a representation in the ego of the whole person constructed in analogy to representations of objects. Hartmann's redefinition may have been, at least in part, a conservative attempt to revise the Freudian system in response to more radical revisions that were flourishing in Britain and would eventuate in the so-called object-relations school of psychoanalysis.

Of great interest in this regard is Fairbairn's (1944) modification of Freud's concept of the ego. Guntrip (1961, p.279) described Fairbairn's ego as "the primary psychic self in its original wholeness, a whole which differentiates into organized structural patterns under the impact of experience of object relationships after birth." With Fairbairn, the detailed considerations of relations to objects began to be more important than the instinctual drives that energized them. The modification of Freud's theory by Fairbairn was criticized by Winnicott (1954), who nonetheless himself proceeded to reshape the traditional theory. Winnicott clearly understood the emergent self of the infant to be related to a holding environment as provided by the mother. The coincidence of the infant's hallucination of anticipated satisfaction with the reality of the gratification supplied by the mother becomes, according to Winnicott, a "moment of illusion" in which the infant experiences himself as omnipotent; this experience becomes the source for the development of a strong and healthy self. Thus Winnicott's moment of illusion was a turn away from Freud's hypothetical moment of hallucinatory satisfaction with its emphasis on frustration as the instigator of development. Many of Winnicott's other insights into the vicissitudes of mother–infant relationships and the development of the self are closely related to Kohut's later formulations and anticipate the direction of Kohut's thinking (cf. Brandchaft, 1986), particularly foreshadowing his interest in what he first came to call the narcissistic personality disorders (Kohut, 1968) and later, the disorders of the self (Kohut & Wolf, 1978).

The narcissistic disorders have in recent years become a much discussed problem in psychoanalysis (Basch, 1986). In previous decades the tremendous discoveries made by Freud in the realm of object libidinal development and its vicissitudes had led to an emphasis on the study and discussion of the psychopathology of the classical psychoneuroses and neurotic characters. Freud's fundamental discoveries in narcissism, its development and its miscarriage, had been duly noted, but were not often followed through to a thorough exploration of the narcissistic disorders—perhaps because the narcissistic neuroses were so unresponsive to psychoanalytic treatment. The often difficult and demanding nature of such patients may also have discouraged analysts from giving the narcissistic disorders and the borderline states and their psychodynamic structure the same kind of searching attention that were given to the more treatable and tractable psychoneuroses. Indeed, Fenichel (1945, p. 574) summarized the prevailing opinion that in the narcissistic neuroses psychoanalysis seems inapplicable, though he pointed out that this "rule" has important exceptions.

However, I would suggest that in addition to these and other difficulties that stood in the way of a more intensive investigation of these narcissistic disorders there were other factors, less scientific and more personal, that made working with narcissistic patients not quite as rewarding. I have in mind particularly the prevailing moral climate of our Judeo-Christian civilization that can sometimes forgive and try to redeem the man who is victim of his passions, whether they be sexual or aggressive, but that finds it very difficult to give a fair hearing to the man who presents himself as smugly superior and arrogantly self-righteous. Freud has influenced us to adopt a slightly more rational attitude toward the failed fate of loving others even when this became manifest by excesses of destructiveness or sexual perversions. But a similarly miscarried love of self was until recently also viewed with moral misgivings and not a fit topic for serious scientists to concern themselves with. Indeed, the biased condemnation that at one time was heaped upon Freud for his attention to the taboo topic of sexuality is reminiscent of contemporary reluctance to examine narcissism and the self because these latter topics are associated with selfishness and being egotistical. Yet, it seems, the time to face our own narcissism has come.

. 2 .

GENERAL ORIENTATION:
THE INNER LIFE OF MAN

Participation in an analysis, whether as analyst or as analysand, is a most palpable enterprise. People who have been analyzed usually know that they have undergone a unique and intense experience. However, when viewed as an activity, psychoanalysis is characterized by an indeterminacy of definition. Both method and theory defy easy classification among the varieties of human endeavors. To talk and write about psychoanalysis requires finding the verbal expressions that can reflect private perceptions into a public domain where they can be shared. It is a job more for a poet than for an objective observer of the processes of nature. Freud himself noted this. It struck him as odd that the case histories he wrote read like short novels and seemed to lack the serious stamp of science (Freud, 1895). Freud, of course, was a highly trained investigator in what today we would call the neurosciences. Though late in life he accepted the award of the Goethe Prize for literature, Freud repeatedly rejected any references to his work as being artistic and thought of such allusions as a form of resistance and repudiation of analysis (Freud, 1920b). Yet the scientific status of psychoanalysis has remained controversial (Grünbaum, 1984). Clearly, a discipline that deals with private perceptual experiences, no matter how systematically and objectively, is in some fundamental ways different from one that deals with publicly verifiable physical phenomena. This difference is important, and it has determined to some extent my way of presenting the theories and practices of psychoanalytic self psychology in this book. For instance, it means that, generally speaking, I cannot define clearly and precisely the concepts and terms that I am using. Clarity of definition must emerge out of usage, which is to say that clinical practice infuses terminology with the meaning that description alone cannot provide. Though at first glance the need for such hands-on acquaintance may appear awkward and unscientific in the conventional sense, it is not an altogether unsatisfactory state of affairs. The dearth of fixed definitions of the verbal kind deters concepts from becoming frozen dogma. Freud found it necessary to repeatedly recast the meaning of even basic terms. After a century of development no standard psychoanalytic theory and practice has emerged in spite of the best efforts of those who have felt uncomfortable with the fluidity that allows for continuous change and progress. It may sound paradoxical, but the psychoanalytic enterprise is still so young, healthy, and vigorous that there is not even agreement yet on what is and what is not psychoanalysis.

Ideally, one learns about psychoanalysis and about psychoanalytic self psychology not by reading, but by experiencing them. Discussions such as the present one, however, are useful if they enrich by helping one to understand and to conceptualize the analytic experience. More importantly, I hope that some readers may be stimulated to seek further analytic experience, whether as analyst or as analysand, to test out for themselves the ideas advanced by self psychology. Making these ideas accessible is my purpose.

Notwithstanding the imprecise nature of psychoanalytic terms, I still find it necessary to present an overview of self-psychological ideas and terminology as a means of easing entry into the subject matter: the clinical experience of self psychology. In addition, a glossary at the end of the book will help to keep from getting lost.

AN OVERVIEW

Human beings are born *pre-adapted* to actively participate in both physical and psychological interactions with the environment, which provide, respectively, for the individuals physical and psychological needs. Both are necessary for survival.

From the beginning, the neonate responds to stimuli with signs indicating the experience of comfort or discomfort. Presumably, at birth, no sense of self can be said to exist, though caregivers address the infant as if indeed he or she were consciously a person. Kohut refers to this phenomenon as the *virtual self* of the infant, in rough analogy to the optical phenomenon of a virtual image. Tremendous strides in infant research during recent years have filled many gaps in our knowledge about early psychological development (Lichtenberg, 1983; Stern, 1985). An integration of these research data with the theories of self psychology is an urgent task.

Apparently, the human tendency to organize experience yields psychological structures that manifest in the subjective experience of things "making sense." Self psychology observes the emergence of a sense of selfhood during the second year of life. It therefore infers the presence of a psychological structure, the *self*. Self psychology is the study of this structure, its subjective manifestations, and its vicissitudes.

The most fundamental finding of self psychology is that the emergence of the self requires more than the inborn tendency to organize experience. Also required are the presence of others, technically designated as *objects*, who provide certain types of experiences that will *evoke* the emergence and maintenance of the self. The perhaps awkward term for these is *selfobject experiences*, usually abbreviated to *selfobjects*. Proper selfobject experiences favor the structural *cohesion* and energic *vigor* of the self; *faulty* selfobject experiences facilitate the *fragmentation* and *emptiness* of the self. Along with food and oxygen, every human being requires age-appropriate selfobject experiences from infancy to the end of life. However, whereas the infant requires the concrete physical presence of the caregiving object as the provider of proper selfobject experiences, the maturely developed adult can maintain the structural integrity of his or her self by selfobject experiences generated in symbolic representations of the original self-evoking experiences.

By taking this just presented outline of basic concepts and terms as an orienting map of psychoanalytic self psychology, the reader will be able to navigate the complex mental states, their pathology, and their treatment, which I deal with later in this book. For the present I will illustrate and elaborate this basic outline of concepts by descriptions that may evoke in the reader a resonance with familiar experiences of his or her own.

EXPERIENCING THE SELF

I am a person, an individual. I think, I feel, I experience. Sometimes I am suffused with energy and with a feeling of well-being and optimism. Sometimes I feel depressed, without much energy, and without the capacity to focus my thinking. At such times I may suffer from aches and pains, my movements are more awkward, perhaps I worry about my health and in general have a low opinion of myself and the world. The future may look bleak; I may be pervaded by a nameless anxiety.

Manifestly, in this brief description, I am pointing primarily to two states of self experience at the opposite poles of a rainbow of self states: at one end, a state of well-being, and at the other, a state of anxious depression. I would guess that most people would find these rough sketches familiar enough from their own experiences. Indeed, I take for granted that I will be understood when I refer to experiencing various states of my self, or when I conjecture about other people's experience of the states of their selfs. Notice that I seem to slip without much concern from talking about myself to talking about my "self," from talking about experiences to talking about states of the self— essentially from a subjective report to a more objectified description of something I assume to exist, as it were, behind my experiences of myself. This is where theory comes in. I am assuming that a psychological structure, my self, is part of a psychological system or organization which gives rise to my experiences.

When I cut myself and bleed, I assume the existence of an injured circulatory structure, part of a circulatory system, that accounts for the bleeding I observe. Experientially, I am usually not very aware of the structure of my circulatory system, especially when it is functioning well. This is also true of my self. But when a structure is malfunctioning, I will experience certain symptoms. I can take my pulse and infer something about the state of my circulation; similarly, I can pay attention to my thoughts and moods and make inferences about what seems to be going on with my self. In this way I can arrive at theories about my self, its structure, its components, its functioning, its development, its relations with itself and with other selfs, and so on. There exist any number of such self theories— everyone naturally develops a self psychology—and they are more or less useful in daily life when dealing with one's own self and the presumed selfs of others.

But observations of one's self by oneself has its limits. I may notice that the presence of certain others always enhances my feeling of well-being. In contrast, the presence of some people generally leaves me feeling disconcerted, to say the least. But the conceptualization of the processes entailed in these observations of myself is another matter. For this purpose I have learned to use the psychoanalytic self psychology developed by Heinz Kohut. Kohut, like Freud before him, was one of those rare psychological geniuses who could take some old and familiar observations, look at them from a fresh point of view, and synthesize an original and systematic approach to observing and reorganizing the psychological data. Borrowing from Kohut's self psychology, I would now label my self-experience of being in a state of well-being as being derived from the *cohesion* of my self. Again, implied in this statement is the theory that the self is a structure; that is, it endures over time and changes comparatively slowly. Therefore, the self has a history—a past, a present, and a future. Clearly, that theoretical proposition is also in harmony with my self-observation. I do experience myself as the same person that I have been for many years and expect to be in the future. No matter how much I have changed and will continue to change, I experience myself as the same person. I of course realize the metaphorical nature of the word "self" as a label for the psychological organization that gives rise to my self experience; and I know that reference to the self's structure, components, and cohesion is also metaphorical. Yet, it is extremely useful to speak in similes and analogies and probably unavoidable, as Freud (1926) said long ago:

> In psychology we can only describe things by the help of analogies [*Vergleichungen*]. There is nothing peculiar in this; it is the case elsewhere as well. But we have constantly to keep changing these analogies, for none of them lasts us long enough. (p. 195)

So returning now to my occasional self experience of being apprehensive, without energy, moody, ill-focused, and disorganized, I might describe this feeling informally as the sense that I am falling apart. The Kohutian term for this state is *fragmentation*, that is, the aspects of one's self-experience seem no longer coordinated or fitting together. Metaphorically, one can conceptualize the structure of the self breaking up into its component fragments. I have observed in my self and in others many instances of feeling fragmented, sometimes more, sometimes less so, and they do not occur in a vacuum. They happen in response to something going on in the surround, or perhaps, to the failure of something to go on there.

Perhaps I am walking down the street and see a friend who passes me by as if I did not exist. It does not seem to matter that the friend was preoccupied and did not see me. Momentarily I am less my self than before. The effect is similar to being asked why I look so bad today. No matter what loving concern may be motivating the compassionate inquiry, suddenly I feel robbed of a piece of my self-image, of a needed confirming response to my presence; and, indeed, self psychology would conceptualize that the missing or faulty response—at any rate, in terms of my present need—is equivalent to a loss of self structure. We would infer that I need something from the milieu around me, a response to me of a particular kind, in order to experience a feeling of well-being. Or, in self-psychological language, my self needs such responses for the completeness and cohesion of its structure. The experience of these self-sustaining responses are called *selfobject experiences*, because they emanate from objects—people, symbols, other experiences—and they are necessary for the emergence, maintenance, and completion of my self. Thus, the theory of psychoanalytic self psychology postulates that selfs come into being and stay whole in consequence of a person's having sustaining selfobject experiences. The self cannot exist as a cohesive structure—that is, cannot generate an experience of well-being—apart from the contextual surround of appropriate selfobject experiences.

Let us look also at some observations that most people who have spent some time with small children have had occasion to make. A small child, of perhaps age two, may be playing contentedly alone with some toys while the mother is busy with something else. Apparently, neither is paying any attention to the other, though an acute observer might catch some quick glances, as if mother and child were each ascertaining the other's presence at intervals. If the mother leaves the room, however, so that the child can no longer see her, the child will probably try to follow her and, if frustrated in this endeavor, will probably start to cry. Under such circumstances, the mother's reappearance, supplemented perhaps by some soothing noises and gestures, will usually restore the child's prior state of well-being.

There are many ways to interpret this sequence of events,[1] but guided by self psychology, I would conceptualize that the mother's absence temporarily deprived the youngster of a needed selfobject experience: that of sensing the mother's active and benevolent inter-

---

1. Among psychoanalytic theoreticians, the conceptualizations of M. Mahler and J. Bowlby are most relevant to these considerations.

est in him or her. Such a selfobject experience confirms the child's subjective sense of self, or, in objective language, this experience, that is, the mother's appropriate responsiveness, supports and sustains the structure and cohesion of the self. One year later, when the child is three or so, the mother might easily leave the room for a while without the child's experiencing any discomfort or threat to its self—as long as the child was still aware of the mother's presence in the house, perhaps by hearing her movements. A few years later, it would probably be possible for mother to leave the house with a brief comment, "I'm going to the store, I'll be right back." Some increased tension—not enough to label it anxiety—might be the extent of the discomfort experienced by the youngster, without any loss of structural integrity of the self. An age-appropriate development of the self has occurred that has changed the form of the needed selfobject experience. The actual physical presence of the caregiving person is still required much of the time, but the intervals of absence can be longer. The child's needs for selfobject experiences have not diminished, but memory and attention span have increased, such that the sustaining effects of the selfobject experience on the self last longer. Also, other experiences have taken the place of some aspects of the child's concrete direct experiences with the caregiver. These may be toys or the familiar surroundings of the home, or siblings, or the good smells emanating from the steak broiling in the oven, or the daily TV fare: All these can have assumed the functions of selfobjects. To the extent that the environment provides selfobject experiences, one may speak of a selfobject ambience consisting of a net of selfobject relationships.[2]

As an adult, one still needs selfobject experiences, though their form has developed significantly beyond those appropriate for a five-year-old. When my own self-esteem is low, I can usually find enhancement by listening to music or by reading. The environment that provides a sustaining selfobject ambience for me includes not only family and friends, but my work and the associations that it fosters. Beyond that, being part of a community and partaking of its culture and values is immensely confirming.

2. Contemporary research on infants has produced a wealth of observations and data that can be interpreted in support of the hypotheses summarized in the selfobject concept (see especially Stern, 1985).

GENERAL COMMENTS ON THE ROLE OF THEORY

Guidance by theory makes it possible to gather usable data from a chaos of perceptions, and theory makes it possible to formulate the data into conceptualizations that lead to rational approaches to diagnosis and treatment. Several levels of theory can be distinguished in psychology. On the most general level there exist sociocultural assumptions that are both conscious and unconscious. For example, when people act contrary to an average expectable range of "normal" behaviors, they are generally thought to "have something wrong with them." The "what" of "what's wrong with you?" may be answered differently by different groups within the larger sphere of Western society. The same "abnormal" behavior may be conceptualized as divergently as possession by evil spirits, hereditary criminality, or neuroticism. Different belief systems are at the root of these divergencies. The belief system known as science has been in the ascendancy in the West for some centuries now and has to a large extent shaped our attitudes toward the natural nonhuman forces in the universe. The successes of the natural sciences have not been matched by the humanistic sciences, and we have yet to find the optimal form for the scientific study of humankind. In this quest, traditional psychoanalysis and its development into self psychology represent significant steps forward.

On a somewhat less general level, there seems to be a high consensus among psychologists that the adult's behavior, in spite of various inherited predispositions, is to a large extent influenced by what he or she experienced as a child. Wordsworth's pithy "The Child is father of the Man" expresses the developmental psychology embedded in modern cultural consciousness. On the other hand, although the childhood roots of many aspects of adult behavior and experience are evident to most thoughtful observers, the patterns of early experience are modified throughout the life history by ongoing interactions with the surround. Adult psychology, therefore, is not merely an adult version of childlike behaviors and feelings, but consists of all the reactions and alterations accumulated over the years and imposed on and amalgamated with the self that emerged during early childhood. Psychoanalytic Self Psychology is a refined and systematic scientific elaboration of such a developmental psychology.

PSYCHOANALYTIC DATA

Freud was an unsurpassed master in the presentation of clinical material. He used his case histories and vignettes as well themes from literature and art to illustrate his ideas. It is not clear whether Freud had more in mind than mere illustration. Perhaps he hoped the narrative data in his case histories had the persuasive power of more precisely defined scientific data. Such an absence of formal precision while relying on demonstrable usage in context may represent an implied recognition of the peculiar scientific status of psychoanalysis. In psychoanalysis we do not deal with the same kind of data on which the physical sciences depend; that is, we do not obtain specifically psychoanalytic data by observing objects in an observational field outside the observer, and, therefore, we cannot easily define either psychoanalytic objects or the observing instruments precisely by recourse to everyday object-related language.

For example, a psychoanalyst might observe an analysand lying on the couch, tensely rigid in posture, speaking with difficulty through teeth that are tightly clenched, in a pinched tone of voice that appears to arise from pushing against tautly stretched vocal cords. The content of what the analysand is saying may express directly some of the thoughts and feelings related to the manner of expression, for example, "I am afraid of him," but it is equally possible that the content may have no obvious relation to what the analysand appears to be experiencing. The tense analysand may be saying, "He is being very kind to me." That is, he may ignore his feelings or even attempt to hide them by talking about something else, "Isn't it a beautiful afternoon?"

What would be specifically psychoanalytic data here? To be sure, all the observations about the analysand's posture, tone of voice, and content of speech would be useful psychological data obtained by the analyst through processing mainly the perceptions of his eyes and ears. However, such processing would not render these observations specifically psychoanalytic data, but merely psychological data that could be obtained by any more or less sophisticated psychological observer. Psychoanalytic data *per se* are obtained by introspections and empathy, and refer to the analysand's inner experiences (Agosta, 1984; Kohut, 1959, 1982; Schwaber, 1984). Thus, by being empathically immersed into his analysand, frequently, over a long period of time and having become familiar with the analysand's history, feelings, thoughts, ideas, worries, and hopes and his mode of experiencing and expressing these, the analyst will gradually acquire a capacity to access the analysand's inner experience: the capacity to be empathically resonating or affectively attuned. Psychoanalytic access to what the patient is experiencing is by empathy.

I discuss empathy as an important tool for data gathering and for the conduct of psychoanalytic treatment more fully in Chapter 3, pp. 34–38. For the present, it is sufficient to stress that the objective-observational data are important data, but not specifically psychoanalytic data; rather, they serve as clues to what the analysand is experiencing, and they evoke *in the analyst* associations, memories, and affects to which he has access by introspection. The trained analyst, guided by his extensive knowledge of himself and of his analysands, gathered over a long period of time, uses awareness of his own introspectively obtained mental state as the springboard for conclusions about the analysand's mental state. This does not mean that the analyst assumes that the analysand's mental state is the same as or similar to his own. But the analyst is able to conclude something about the analysand's current inner experience from what is being evoked in his own mental state by his interaction with the analysand, from his self-knowledge, from his knowledge of the analysand, from previous experiences with this and other analysands, and, perhaps, also from numerous unconscious clues. This is the process of what Freud called *Einfuehlung*, to feel oneself into another—what we call empathy—and it yields the specifically psychoanalytic data. These data lead one to talk about being able to "understand" the analysand, and, in conjunction with explanatory theoretical concepts, one can arrive at hypothetical explanations of what the analysand is experiencing or, as we like to call them when we communicate them to the analysand, interpretations. The observational field from which the analyst obtains these psychoanalytic data par excellence are the subjectively experienced mental states of the analytic team, that is, both analyst and analysand.

Definitions in psychoanalysis, therefore, are of a different nature than in the physical sciences. For one thing, in contrast to the phenomena defined by the physical sciences, they cannot be subjected to mathematical operations. Instead of describing events in a three-dimensional world, the terms we use point metaphorically and evocatively to psychological experiences by the use of connotation and analogy. These refer to subjective mental states through their content, allusions, and associated affects. The perceptions designated by these terms and their subjectively derived definitions are themselves subject to distortions. That is why such terms as "hostility" or "love" or "self" or "transference" defy all efforts to pin them down with precision, earning us the contempt of some of the "hard" scientists among us.

DISSENTING VIEWS OF THE ANALYTIC PROCESS

Not all psychoanalysts conceptualize their working methods in the manner I have just described. Some claim to work and apparently do work in a different manner because they deem empathic data to be unreliable. The biased influences emanating from the personality of the analyst may distort the obtained empathic data and, therefore, the use of empathic data is thought to be unscientific. But in any scientific data collection, biases may slip in and the various sciences have developed methods for keeping these distorting intrusions to a minimum. Rigorous analytic and scientific training in combination with self-knowledge gained through personal analysis and supervision serves the same controlling purpose in psychoanalysis.

The main source of controversy here is that we seem to have two different ways of conceptualizing what we mean by data in psychoanalysis. On the one hand, there is the point of view that in order for data to be acceptable as scientific they must be obtained in ways that are consensually verifiable and replicable—as is, of course, true for the natural sciences. For some psychoanalysts, that means making very careful observations of the analysand's demeanor, dress, behavior, organized speech, and free associations, both as to content and form as well as to tone of voice and inflection, and so forth. Usually, taking notes is deemed sufficient for recording, but videotapes have been used to increase reliability. From this material, together with the available extra-analytic data, such as the case history and so forth, and guided by psychoanalytic theory, some make inferences as to the analysand's intrapsychic conflicts and attempt to formulate the intrapsychic conflict in psychodynamic terms. Such analysts claim that empathy does not play a decisive role in the way they come to conclusions about their analysands; thus they believe their methods are more objectively scientific and less an arbitrary projection of the analyst's biases and countertransference reactions onto the patient.

The contrasting methodology shifts the position of the analyst as observer away from the readily accessible overt appearance of the analysand, away from his observable behavior, and away from the verbalized content of speech. Instead, the analyst as participant-observer posits himself "inside" the experiencing analysand. The major emphasis is on attempting to gain access to the analysand's subjective experience. To achieve this means to include, in *addition* to all the data that can be obtained by an outside observer, the analyst's vicarious introspection into the analysand—in other words, to include the analysand's presumed introspection. Empathic immersion also means that all the data observed from the outside are reassessed and recast into experiential terms from the analysand's presumed point of view. Indeed, Kohut's (1977, p. 306) statement that the very idea of human mental life is "unthinkable" without the ability to know by means of empathy, as elaborated by Agosta (1984, p. 48), becomes the cornerstone for the possibility of constituting the field of psychoanalysis. The empathic vantage point becomes the organizer for all observations made. The analyst attempts to put himself into the analysand's shoes, so to speak, but not by asking himself what he, the analyst, would experience under these circumstances, but by asking himself what this particular patient—about whom he knows so much—would be apt to experience in this context. Empathic data collection leads the analyst to understand what the analysand experiences. The analyst then processes this understanding by way of some psychoanalytic theoretical conceptualization that explains the experience as he understands it. Understanding plus explaining add up to an interpretation. An illustration follows.

During the second year of her analysis, a young mother reported that her own mother, who had been comatose for several weeks, had died. As a child, this analysand's relationship to her mother had been one of intense ambivalence, because the mother, in addition to being almost constantly critical of the daughter's behavior, also said on repeated occasions that she really did not like her daughter and predicted she would come to a bad end. Fortunately, the daughter got along famously with her father—until the latter left the family, divorced, and remarried. Mother and daughter, both left behind, patched up a fragile truce that was often punctured by hostile outbursts from either. The mother had had a similarly hostile relationship with her own mother, and she frequently accused the analysand of being a tramp like the girl's grandmother. When the analysand arrived for her first session after her mother's death, she talked about her mother's prolonged illness and death with some sadness. Of course, she added matter-of-factly, she felt a sense of relief that her mother's suffering had ended. She then reported a dream in which a man was staring at her bare legs.

My own inner experience while listening to her, however, was not in resonance with her apparent sadness nor with the heavy mood that one might expect to emanate from a mourning person. Instead she had evoked in me an almost flirtatious impulse. I concluded, empathically tuning into her inner state, that, indeed, she was not experiencing much mourning, sadness, or depression, but was in a playful frame of mind, though she gave no outward sign of the latter; my inner response was the only clue. I then noticed that she was not wearing stockings that day, which was unusual for this usually well-dressed woman. Was this slight deterioration of her dress evidence for some depressive phenomenon, or was it a slightly seductive display of her legs to evoke an admiring response that she might experience as sustaining to her self-esteem, or was it both? Introspecting into my affective resonance, I felt from my reaction that she was feeling flirtatious rather than depressed. Her protestations of sadness, I concluded, were a *pro forma* conventional response. Her flirtatiousness was evident and, I reasoned, was being used defensively against becoming aware of the deeply painful feelings of loss with which she was unable to cope at the moment. Using my empathic perception of her inner experience together with what I knew about her history, I interpreted her behavior as her attempt to show me that she was reacting properly to her mother's death by telling me she was sad; but, I continued, the death had stirred up such intensely painful feelings of loss that she had to deny them by feeling playful and by evoking admiring attention to her self, much as she had obtained her father's attention during childhood when her mother had spurned her. Her bare legs, as well as a more general lack of attention to her dress, seemed related both to the underlying depressive affect associated with the loss of her mother and to the yearning for attention. The interpretation was followed by a more pronounced depressive affect. A flare-up in somatic symptoms on the subsequent day appeared to confirm that interpretation.

This patient could not accept the pain and depression associated with the loss of mother without having a supportive selfobject experience to strengthen her self first. She therefore hid the pain and depression from herself by covering these affects with a flirtatious exterior, both in behavior and dream. Empathically I recognized this behavior, as well as her not-quite-successful attempt at matter-of-factness, as a superficial defense against the deeper painful affects. By explaining this connection to her, that is, by making an interpretation, I helped her experience me as interested, without her needing to be seductive or playful to keep me interested, and genuinely concerned with her rather than with some superficial and conventionally stylized expression of mourning. This experience of me was for her a strengthening selfobject experience that made it possible to let herself also experience the full impact of the sadness, depression, and mourning. In this effect on her my interpretation I would give the highest priority to her total experience of me and my attitude toward her and less importance to the precise verbal content of the interpretation. However, it was the calm reasoning and reassuring (not criticizing her for flirtatiousness) content of the interpretation to her which implied my strength and my continued nonexploitative (in contrast to her father) interest in her, that allowed her to have the sustaining total selfobject experience. In general, a deepening of the analysis as evidenced by the coming to the surface of self-awareness of previously repressed or denied material can be taken as a confirmation of the proper functioning of the interpretative process.

It should be added that, of course, the interpretive inferences that I drew from my empathic perceptions and from other knowledge may well have been incorrect (though they seem confirmed by the further course of the analysis). Here I am merely demonstrating steps in the empathic–interpretive process.

· 3 ·

BASIC CONCEPTS OF
SELF PSYCHOLOGY

INTRODUCTION

In the previous chapter, I began to describe some of the basic observations that a person can make about his or her inner life and that of others. I tried to show how these observations can lead to theoretical inferences about a presumed psychological structure, *the self,* and about a presumed psychological organization, *the self-selfobject system.*[1] The conceptualizations of the relationships within this self–selfobject system are known as the theory of self psychology. Historically, self psychology emerged out of the practice of psychoanalysis. The theoretical framework Kohut propounded represents a far-reaching reconceptualization of the underpinnings of psychoanalytic theory and practice. The purpose of this chapter is to provide a general introduction to the concepts and methods of self psychology, as these have been elaborated by Kohut and his followers.[2] A more detailed examination of the basic concepts will follow in Chapter 4.

Kohut was influenced relatively little by the other main psychoanalytic contributors to the post-Freudian era, though he was conversant with both the traditional classic and neo-Freudian literature. Working independently, Kohut developed a systematic psychoana-

1. To infer the existence of a psychological structure, the self, as part of a presumed psychological system is roughly on the same theoretical level as the inference, from all kinds of observations, of the existence of electrons as part of a presumed system of electromagnetic phenomena.

2. The pertinent works include Atwood & Stolorow (1984), Basch (1983), Goldberg (1978, 1980, 1983, 1985), Kohut (1971, 1977, 1978, 1984, 1985), Kohut & Wolf (1978), Lichtenberg & Kaplan (1983), Ornstein & Ornstein (1985), Stepansky & Goldberg (1984), Stolorow & Lachmann (1980), M. Tolpin (1971), P. Tolpin (1980), Wolf (1976b, 1980b, 1982), and Wolf, Gedo, & Terman (1972).

lytic approach that was original, comprehensive, and innovative while based on the basic principles of psychoanalysis as formulated by Freud.[3]

In order to comprehend Kohut's self-psychological approach without the distortions imposed by one's prior commitments to alternate points of view, it is necessary, temporarily, to set aside these prior notions. To grasp Kohut, one must listen open-mindedly, without wondering about id, ego, and superego, or about drives, instinctual conflicts, and resistances. These concepts are useful at the proper time, but they should be temporarily displaced to the periphery. Instead, for a full appreciation of Kohut's theoretical and clinical achievement, the *self* and its *selfobjects* must be made the center of concern and the focus of one's conceptualizing.

Most of the patients that seek help today from mental health professionals—from psychoanalysts, psychiatrists, psychologists, social workers, group therapists, counseling services—suffer from what self psychologists have come to call *disorders of the self*. It is much less common today to see a patient who presents him- or herself with the typical symptoms of one of the classical psychoneuroses as described by Freud. Thirty years ago, when I first entered the private practice of psychiatry in a big city, I still had patients who came for help with clearly delineated neurotic symptoms, such as a conversion hysteria or obsessive–compulsive rituals. Psychiatrists treated patients with disabling hand-washing compulsions, and there were other patients who had suddenly lost their voice or who suffered changed or lost sensations or the use of part of their limbs (hysterical paralyses, paresthesias, and anesthesias). Often these patients responded to psychoanalytic treatment or to psychoanalytically oriented psychotherapy. I understand that occasionally these classical psychoneurotic syndromes are still seen by physicians working with more rural populations.

I myself, however, have not seen in many years such a once-familiar type of patient with classical neurotic symptom patterns. I gather that this is also true of my colleagues. It would be of the

3. Some of the ideas introduced earlier into psychoanalysis by the British psychoanalysts that have come to be known as the object relations school are very similar to Kohut's concerns and concepts. Still, they are not the same, and it is Kohut's unique achievement to have developed the "subjective" point of view into a comprehensive psychology.

greatest interest to investigate in detail the changing patterns of psychological symptomatology. Do changes in our cultural ambience account for this shift in the patterns of morbidity? It has been postulated that changing styles of child rearing together with changing size, composition, and distribution of responsibilities within family relationships would emerge as the cause for the observed movement toward a preponderance of self disorders (cf. Kohut, 1977, pp. 269–271). It is plausible, for example, that in the extended upper middle-class family of Freud's Vienna, the child was not neglected, but overstimulated in an ambience of hypersexuality precisely because the mores of the day favored that sex be hush-hush and illicit, not to be talked about but enjoyed on the sly. The degree of preoccupation with sexuality in those days of Victorian puritanism can be gathered by recalling that in some of the best houses piano legs were draped with skirts so as to be neither overstimulating nor offensive. Today, in contrast, little remains hidden about sexuality. Furthermore, and this is probably of the greatest importance, the extended family of aunts, uncles, cousins, cooks, maids, governesses, and so forth has mostly shrunk to the core family of siblings and parents, none of whom are at home enough to be easily and generously available to the youngsters. The key person for needed selfobject responsiveness, the mother, is much more likely to have to go out to work, and, at any rate, to be more overworked and harrassed by the multiplicity of demands made on her than her grandmother was. Institutional substitutes such as schools and day care centers have yet to demonstrate that they can provide a child with sufficient stimulation and psychological nourishment, that is, with appropriate selfobject experiences, to avoid the child's feeling uncared for and unresponded to. In contemporary society, therefore, the shrinking importance of the family results in a gradual impoverishment of the self-sustaining aspects of the selfobject experiences that the child has. This may be one explanation for the apparently increasing morbidity of narcissistic disorders, that is, disorders of the self. One also wonders whether the increasing seriousness of drug abuse among young people and the steadily increasing suicide rate during the last two decades could be related to the shifting child rearing patterns that are deficient in self-sustaining and self-supporting experiences.

Some people have always suffered from narcissistic disorders. The special attention contemporary psychotherapists pay them now in contrast to previous decades is not only a consequence of the greater morbidity but is also the result of better understanding of the problem, which encourages interest among therapists. It is a common tendency to ignore or reject, that is, to disavow the sources of unpleasantness when one feels helpless to deal with them. Such was the position of psychoanalysis *vis-à-vis* the so-called "narcissistic neuroses." They were deemed difficult, if not impossible, to treat psychoanalytically. Psychoanalysts usually did not accept patients with psychoses or psychotic-like conditions for psychoanalysis, although valiant attempts were made to modify classical treatment techniques, especially for the psychotherapy of so-called borderline patients. The emergence of a psychology of the self has made it possible to understand and therefore to treat many of these formerly untreatable self disorders with a reasonable expectation of achieving significant improvement. As experience with severely regressed patients grows, so does the empathic understanding of their inner life. Thus, there is reasonable hope that further improvement in treatability by self-psychological analytic techniques will gradually accrue, perhaps not excluding even psychotic patients (cf. Galatzer-Levy, 1988).

The following illustrative vignette will elaborate what is meant by the concepts self and selfobject experience: Imagine a speaker in front of a group of respected colleagues. As he stands there, he feels pretty good, but slightly apprehensive. How will they receive what he has to say? He tells them what he has on his mind and they listen, more or less attentively. That makes him feel that he is being heard and responded to. As a result, he feels good, more sure of himself. In other words, his self-esteem is enhanced. And, perhaps, the audience will think that this fellow has it "all together." To put this a little more theoretically, apparently he needs this responsiveness because his self, a psychological structure as we see it, needs certain sustaining psychological responses from its surroundings in order to remain cohesive and vigorous. These self-sustaining responses are performed for the self by objects, and we call these needed responses *selfobject responses*, or, more precisely, *selfobject experiences* of the object.

But suppose, instead, that the audience is getting a little bored with this speaker's presentation. Perhaps the speaker is noticing a lot of yawning or stretching and restlessness in the room and that some people are beginning to walk out. What would happen to the speaker as a result? Probably he would begin to feel rather uncomfortable, a little distracted, and then he might become unsure of himself; perhaps he would begin to stumble over his words, or he would lose his place, or his voice would give out or he might blush or break out in a sweat. One need not give a detailed description of what it is like when one suddenly feels unresponded to, disconnected from one's surroundings. Everyone has experienced this at times and knows that the unconnected state is most unpleasant. We spoke of this unhappy state earlier as the feeling that one is "falling apart." To conceptualize this, one might say that the speaker's self had fragmented because of insufficient selfobject responses. However, the terms "to fragment" or "fragmentation" are easily misunderstood, because they are derived from introspective–empathic experiences. In the example just presented, one could also say—in terminology that is a step removed from experience-near observations and corresponds more closely to traditional experience-distant observations—that there had been some regression with some disorganization of the self because of insufficient self-sustaining selfobject experiences. The latter are needed to sustain the solid cohesion of the self.

But let us get back to the self that I have made the center of attention. The self may be defined as that psychological structure which makes its presence evident by providing one with a healthy sense of self, of self-esteem and well-being. It seems that the essence of the self is elusive, very much as the essence of an electron is elusive. All we can really know about these structures are their manifestations, that is, the phenomena to which they give rise. Even the quality of being a psychological structure means no more than that the self can be shown to have a history that is, as already noted, a past, a present, a future, and that over this history certain aspects of the self change only very slowly, if at all. Structure simply means stability over time. This stability can be lost, gradually or suddenly, and there may be rapid changes in function and manifestation, such as an altered sense of self or a lost feeling of well-being. We conceptualize in these cases of structural change that structure has been lost or altered. Thus, we talk about cohesive selfs and fragmented selfs. But, clearly, as I have indicated, these are metaphors for introspected experiences. Psychoanalytic data are derived from subjective experiences and therefore essentially private. To think, talk, and write about psychoanalytic data requires that these experiences be conceptualized in a communicable and objectified language. In the present discourse, therefore, the reader has to follow my constant oscillations between references to experiences and references to objectified conceptualizations that are derived from these experiences.

The self is not a new discovery. The concept precedes psychoanalysis. Indeed, as already mentioned, psychoanalytic psychology until recently did not pay much attention to the self. Among other reasons for this neglect was the felt urgency to investigate those psychological constellations that had been newly discovered by Freud, especially the conflict-laden sexual drives and their vicissitudes. The study of the latter had to proceed in the face of stubborn resistance both from within each individual and from the moralistic society outside the individual. Therefore, any deviation from Freud's courageous program to investigate instinctual drives, conflicts, and defenses was suspect as a probable manifestation of a hidden or well-disguised resistance. Morally speaking, furthermore, any focus on the self coupled with a concern for the self's well-being apparently looks selfish. As already discussed in Chapter 1 to be called egotistical or labeled narcissistic is, in our Judeo-Christian culture, not a compliment. Yet, one would think, such moralistic biases have no place in investigative endeavors. One may hope that reasonable people will consider it legitimate to talk about and to study narcissism without any pejorative connotations.

THE DEPENDENCE ON A SELFOBJECT MATRIX

The observation that the self cannot exist for long in a psychological vacuum is a finding that is not easily accepted. The very emergence and maintenance of the self as a psychological structure depends on the continuing presence of an evoking–sustaining–responding matrix of selfobject experiences. This discovery heralds the end of another cherished illusion of Western man, namely the illusory goal of independence, self-sufficiency, and free autonomy. Clinically, the phenomenon of dependence on a sustaining selfobject matrix is demonstrable in practically every analysand: Once a selfobject transference has become established, any disruption of the continuity of the bond between analyst and analysand is experienced as a threat. Almost invariably one can observe that holidays, vacations, or other absences for most any reason are accompanied by symptoms of regression, and sometimes fragmentation. These phenomena cut across diagnostic categories and appear to represent a basic characteristic of the constitution of self structure. Disruptions in the continuity of the sustaining selfobject experience result in symptoms characteristic of disruptions of the continuity of the self. Outside the clinical situation one may observe analogous phenomena. For instance, creative people frequently depend on the presence of some other person or persons—or, sometimes, some object that symbolizes the presence of the other—for the exercise of their creative skills and talents. Presumably it is the selfobject experience entailed in these relationships that strengthens the self sufficiently to be able to realize these skills productively. Kohut designated this phenomenon the *transference of creativity* (Kohut 1976). Among political figures, for example, the Prussian statesman Bismarck had insomnia that was "cured" by the mere presence of his physician sitting at his bedside until Bismarck had fallen asleep (Kohut, 1984, pp. 19-20). I would wonder whether the closeness of President Wilson to Col. House and that of President Roosevelt to Harry Hopkins were similar needed selfobject experiences that allowed these men to function at optimal capacity. Among artists, the study of Picasso by M. Gedo reveals the close connection between selfobject experience and artistic creation, as exemplified by the mutually self-sustaining attachment of Picasso and Braque (Gedo, 1980, pp. 84-86). Analogous relationships can be found among writers. The German poet Schiller was reported to be unable to write unless he had a rotten apple in his desk drawer. Regrettably, I have no information to speculate on how such a dead fruit acquired a selfobject meaning for Schiller. However, our studies of Virginia Woolf (Wolf & Wolf, 1979) strongly suggest that her husband, Leonard, performed the selfobject functions that permitted Virginia to have the strength to face the emotional upheaval attending the writing and publishing of her self-revealing novels.

Thus, self psychology strikes deeply at a politico-religious value system in which the self-made individual is the ideal. We now have a deeper appreciation of our inescapable embeddedness in our environment. Human development is inseparable from the surrounding environment and cannot be studied in isolation. The psychoanalytic study of the individual inevitably, via self psychology, becomes not the study of the person-in-vacuo but of the person in his or her surround, i.e., the study of the self and its selfobjects as a subjective, experiential phenomenon.

In summary, self psychology (or, perhaps, more precisely, self-object psychology or the psychology of selfobject experiences) is concerned with those vicissitudes of the experience of selfhood that we can talk about using the metaphor of the self. Apparently, it is a characteristic attribute of the human psyche to organize itself so that it experiences the "I am I" as a unified and historically continuous self. Loss of this organization, that is, loss of the sense of selfhood, can be the occasion for the greatest panic and horror.

THE CLINICAL ORIGIN OF SELF PSYCHOLOGY

Kohut derived his new ideas not from theoretical speculations, but from clinical experience in the analysis of what were at that time still called psychoneurotic patients. It was stalemates in the analysis of certain patients that forced him to reconsider his diagnoses and his responses to these patients. To be sure, Freudian theory had been challenged on many grounds before the emergence of self psychology. But it would appear that alteration of the classical framework to accommodate the clinical findings does not guarantee a significant alteration of clinical approach. Many analysts, of course, have always been tactful and sensitive to their patient's needs for a therapeutic alliance and avoided the harshly unresponsive ambience that resulted from an overly strict application of the rule of abstinence. But the emphasis usually remained on technical neutrality and on the concept of unconscious conflict, which required confrontative interpretation. Kohut was forced by his clinical experiences to recognize that the classical approach did not work in some of his so-called "neurotic" patients who were not obviously narcissistic, borderline, or psychotic. When these patients consistently rejected his interpretation of their libidinal and aggressive conflicts or their defenses against these, he decided to stop calling their refusal a resistance and began to let them tell him how they saw and experienced themselves. He noticed that his shift from an implicitly adversarial stance to an explicitly empathically attuned one resulted in the relief of acute symptoms. From this he developed the fundamental insight that the cohesiveness of their self experience was central to the analytic task with these patients. Further, he saw that the vicissitudes of his patient's experience of him—what today we would call the selfobject experience—was, for better or worse, the most powerful ingredient in the therapeutic process. From that beginning Kohut developed his theories about empathy and about selfobject psychology.

THE BIPOLAR SELF

Because the discovery of the selfobject experiences out of which the self emerges seemed initially to point to two main types of selfobject experiences, that is, to the mirroring experiences and to the idealizing experiences, Kohut conceptualized the emerging self as having a *bipolar* structure (see Chapter 4, p. 50*ff.*). By that he meant that during the structural organization of these experiences they became clustered into two structural locations, according to their mirroring or idealizing character. Thus, the emerging self structure could be thought to have two poles. The pole that precipitates out of the mirroring experiences therefore becomes the locus of the need to be confirmed; the basic ambitions for power and success emanate from it. The other pole precipitates out of idealizing experiences and harbors the basic idealized goals. An intermediate area of basic talents and skills are activated by a *tension-arc* that establishes itself between ambitions and ideals.

> The patterns of ambitions, skills and goals; the tensions between them; the program of action that they create; and the activities that strive toward a realization of this program are all experienced as continuous in space and time—they are the self, an independent center of initiative, an independent recipient of impressions. (Kohut & Wolf, 1978, p. 414)

HOW SELF PSYCHOLOGY HAS MODIFIED CLASSICAL PSYCHOANALYSIS

Innate versus Environmental

Classical Freudian psychoanalysis is a psychology of intrapsychic conflict. Basically, it sees the root of motivation in innate biological factors, the so-called instincts. The effects of the environment are mediated secondarily through psychic structures, such as the super-ego. Neo-Freudian schools developed an interpersonal psychology that stresses instead the direct influence of the environment; motivation is shaped by the individual's relation to objects during the formative years. Self psychology takes a position that tries to avoid bias in favor of either biological or environmental influence. The organism, that is, the neonate, is born with certain potentials that are his biological heritage. However, it is interaction with the environment that will evoke some of these potentials and bring them into development, whereas others are left to atrophy or may even be destroyed. Self psychology, like Freudian theory, is focused on the intrapsychic experience of individuals—the selfobject experience—but attempts to be as much aware of the environmental conditions that shape the selfobject experience; it also attempts with the help of the developmental psychology, to delineate the ever-changing age-appropriate selfobject needs of the individual. In classical psychoanalysis, the biological needs,—the inherent instinctual drives—are explicitly described, whereas the environmental contribution to the individual's psychological structure are only implicitly recognized. In self psychology, the reverse is true: The importance of the selfobject environment as a decisive influence on the central selfobject experience is explicitly conceptualized, whereas the equally essential inherent need of the individual for stimuli to organize his inner life, his subjective experience, into a cohesively structured configuration, has been only implicit.

Curiosity and Stimulus Hunger

Like Kohut, the observers of mothers/infant behavior stress neither the biological nor the environmental roots of motivation. They see the neonate born with multiple potentials, some of which develop at an inborn rate, others that develop as evoked by environmental stimuli. Babies have an inborn curiosity and stimulus hunger that leads them to explore their surroundings unless they have been traumatized. These explorations take place as long as the child experiences itself as embedded in an ambience of warmly responsive care. In the absence of such an ambience, the child will be distressed and cease its exploratory behavior.[4]

----

4. For contemporary psychoanalytic surveys of the findings of infant research, see Lichtenberg (1983) and Stern (1985).

Nature versus Nurture

Because Freud thought that the innate drives relentlessly push for discharge, that is, for gratification, he saw organisms as relentlessly attempting to get from the environment the objects they require for drive discharge. As a result, the environment is necessarily understood to be in an adversary relation to the organism.

Self-psychological theory has not directly attempted to examine and explain the biological substrate that would have to be present for the observed psychological phenomena to occur. However, it is implicit in the theory of the self and its development that there exists in the human organism a tendency to organize experience in such a way as to lead to the emergence of consciousness, to the emergence of a sense of personhood (or selfhood), and to the creation of affects that communicate aspects of the inner states of the self to the self and to others. Affects and appetites guide the self's exploration of its surroundings.

Data: Observing from Outside versus Inside

It is useful to divide psychological data into two categories. Observations of the psychological relationships between objects in a field made by an observer stationed outside that field are analogous to the observations of other relationships between objects as they are made by the natural sciences. Thus, in psychology, data can be obtained by observation from the outside, that is, *extrospectively*, as in the natural sciences. In this way one can observe behavior, including verbal behavior, such as speech. Most of the data and findings in the various branches of academic and social psychology are of this type and resemble the way of working of the natural scientists.

In psychology one can also observe inside oneself how one feels, thinks, and experiences, particularly as to affects and attitudes, that is, *introspectively*. By sensing oneself into another's experience, that is, by *vicarious introspection*, one can come to some conclusions about what another person's experience is likely to be. Data obtained by vicarious introspection (= empathy) can be combined with extrospective data to get a more complete picture of the psychological world in depth. By definition, psychoanalytic data must contain an aspect of empathic data. Psychological data—for example, objective descriptions of behavior that do not include the data of subjective experience—are not psychoanalytic data.

Empathy

I have already mentioned that empathy is one of the basic concepts of selfobjects psychology. Some further discussion is indicated. Empathy has a triple function—it defines the depth psychological field, it is a process of data collection, and it is a self-sustaining experience, for the analysand.

The Defining Function

The two types of data in psychology—extrospective data and introspective data—are obtained from different observational fields: extrospective data from the field external to the observer, introspective data from the field internal to the observer, that is, from within. Most of scientific and academic psychology is concerned with the field external to the observer, in analogy to the natural sciences. The field internal to the observer, where data is accessible by introspection and by empathy, is defined as the field of depth psychology. Psychoanalysis is the depth psychology *par excellence* and, as such, it is defined by its method of data collection. However, this does not mean that psychoanalysis can do without extrospective data. By definition, psychoanalysis is the depth psychological science that combines extrospective data with introspectively and empathically derived data. Without empathy there can be no psychoanalytic data and consequently no psychoanalytic science. Empathy thus has a defining function in the construction of psychoanalytic theories.

The Processing Function

A *processing function* of empathy is to obtain the kind of data that are characteristic for psychoanalysis. Psychoanalysis uses various types of data or information about analysands in analogy with other psychologies. Such data may include direct observations, especially of behavior, particularly verbal behavior, as well as other relevant knowledge about the analysand—personal history, family history, the history of his analysis, and the like. However, all these data, though used by psychoanalysis, are not, strictly speaking, psychoanalytic data, because they refer only to the analyst's observations of the analysand as an object. Because psychoanalysis is concerned with the inner experience of individuals, the essential psychoanalytic data must refer to an individual's private experience. But access to private experience is available only by introspection into one's self. Access to the inner experience of others is problematic. For the psychoanalyst to have some ideas about an analysand's inner experience, he must sense it by putting himself, imaginatively, into another's experience: that is, by vicarious introspection. There are clues that can be perceived which allow one to make good educated guesses about another's experience. "He that has eyes to see and ears to hear may convince himself that no mortal can keep a secret. If his lips are silent, he chatters with his fingertips; betrayal oozes out of him at every pore" (Freud, 1905a, pp. 77-78). Many of these clues are unconsciously perceived and probably represent some sort of subliminal affective communication. Freud mentioned turning one's unconscious toward the unconscious of the patient. Although it is not possible to describe precisely the mechanisms by which such affective communications are transmitted, we do know that the process of empathy, of obtaining data by vicarious introspection, becomes more reliable with experience and is trainable. This proceeds very much in analogy to training other perceptions. For example, a fledgling microscopist will see nothing but a turmoil of dots, lines, smudges, and colors when first looking through the microscope at a thin slice of body tissue. Some months later, the same microscopist, now trained and experienced, will see an altogether different image: Instead of the chaos previously seen, he now will recognize an organized structure consisting of cells, membranes, nuclei, and so forth, and he will be able to recognize whether he is looking at a piece of healthy or diseased tissue. Similarly, the fledgling psychotherapist will not have a very clear idea about his patient's private experiences when listening to the turmoil pouring out of a desperately upset human being. Yet the same therapist, some months or years later, after training and experience, will be able to detect the nuances of rage or shame or excitement, of guilt and anxiety, and so forth, when listening to the emotional chaos that pours out. Empathic observations, like microscopic, or radiological, or observations obtained through CT scans or Magnetic Resonance Imaging, depend on trained capacities for perception and interpretation. Surprisingly, this is so even for basic visual perceptions. A person who has been functionally blind since childhood because of corneal opacities will not suddenly be able to "see" objects when these opacities are surgically removed. Rather, it will take weeks or longer before this individual will have learned to organize the visual sensory perceptions of colors and forms into recognizable objects. Like the more familiar five senses, empathy must be "learned."

In this connection, it is interesting to note that one's empathic capacities are partially determined by the context in which one is working. For example, most psychoanalysts have developed a significant capacity for empathic perceptivity with respect to a patient's inner life. Yet the same analyst may well be insensitive to the inner feelings of others in his personal life, outside the familiar confines of his consulting room. This phenomenon calls for research that might reveal information about the conditions favoring empathic perceptions. This would be a useful contribution for the training of psychotherapists.

The Self-Sustaining Function

Knowing that one is understood by another makes one feel better. A person's sense of self is enhanced by the knowledge that another person understands his inner experience—that is, is aware of that inner experience and is responding to it with warmly colored positive affects. This phenomenon can easily be observed by paying close attention to one's inner state introspectively or by empathically getting in touch with another's inner experience. These empirical observations are so fundamental and universal that usually they are taken for granted. One might speculate informally that being understood by another means that the other is unmistakably interested in one and thereby affirming one's self. Using the concepts of self psychology, one might formulate such affirmation as a mirroring selfobject experience. The psychoanalyst who obtains data from his analysand by attempting to listen empathically, by trying to be in tune through vicarious introspection, will, therefore, as a by product of this listening activity, strengthen the cohesion of the analysand's self and increase the analysand's self-esteem and feeling of well-being. Empathic listening has a beneficial effect regardless of the content of the data obtained and in spite of an analyst's errors in grasping the analysand's experience correctly. Therefore, we can speak of a *sustaining-the-analysand's-self function* of empathy.

Patients are commonly upset and anxious or depressed when they start treatment. In the majority of cases one can notice that they begin to feel better when the therapist will listen attentively without interrupting except for a clarifying question now and then. More generally, the initial resistant phase of treatment is frequently followed by a period of a "harmonious" selfobject relationship when the patient feels relatively good, the symptoms have receded somewhat, and the initial tension seems to have drained out of the relationship. This does not indicate any basic improvement in the patient's condition, but is dependent on experiencing a relationship with an empathically attuned selfobject, the therapist. In the past, this phenomenon has been variously referred to as a "transference cure" or as evidence of a good therapeutic alliance. Self psychologically, we conceptualize that the empathic intuneness allows the patient's self to use the therapist as a selfobject that is experienced as part of its own self structure. The patient's self is thus strengthened and experiences itself as more cohesive with an increased sense of well-being.

Empathy is a relatively neutral activity, in that it aims to understand whatever is going on in the other without major participation in the other's experience. To be more precise, "neutral" here means that the therapist maintains sufficient emotional distance to keep his judgment from being clouded by his feelings. Neutrality does not exclude friendliness, nor should the therapist hesitate to see things from the patient's side, that is, from the patient's biased point of view. Nonparticipation simply means that the therapist does not suffer or enjoy along with the patient. Still, here again we must qualify: The therapist has to partake minimally in the patient's feelings, enough to know what it is that the patient is experiencing. Perhaps, this "sampling" of the patient's experience comes close to the signal function of affects that have long been studied by psychoanalysis. By contrast, sympathy is an activity in which the sympathizer fully shares the other's feeling state. When one sympathizes with someone's bereavement, one feels the other's emotion, for example, sadness or grief, and communicates that participation. Empathizing with someone's bereavement means that one fully understands what the other person is experiencing—perhaps one has experienced similar affects oneself—but one is not experiencing them now beyond "picking up on" what the other is feeling, and one is not sharing the other's suffering.

Empathic data can be used for someone's benefit, as in the best of psychotherapy and psychoanalysis, or to someone's detriment. A detrimental use of empathic information might be found in advertising or certain types of sales presentations. For example, a person's hunger for certain inner experiences may be empathically detected and used to sell him something that he neither needs nor should buy, such as intoxicants to an addiction-prone person, and the like.

As already mentioned psychoanalytic data obtained through the psychoanalytic method are ordered differently when guided by the theories of psychoanalytic self psychology than when guided by traditional psychoanalytic theories. In traditional psychoanalysis, these data are organized around the basic concept of drives in conflict. In self psychology, data are organized around a concept of the self in its imperative need to become and remain a cohesive structure as it gives meaningful expression to itself through enacting an intrinsic program. Since the self, in order to stay structurally intact, must be embedded in a matrix of sustaining relationships with selfobjects—that is, selfobject experiences—the vicissitudes of self-object relations become the focus of interest both for the study of the etiology of disorders of the self and for the therapeutic interventions made to ameliorate these disorders.

The Self

That part of the personality which confers the sense of selfhood and which is evoked and sustained by a constant supply of responsiveness from the functioning of selfobjects—thus providing a continuous matrix of selfobject experiences—we call the *self*. Metaphorically, we think of the self as a structure because, like a structure, the self changes only very slowly. Like all structures, we can think of the self as made of parts that either fit well together, as it were, as if well-glued, or can fall apart easily. Therefore, as noted, we speak sometimes of a self that is cohesive, which means put together well, and at other times, of a self that is fragile and easily fragments.

Selfobject Experiences

If a person is to feel well—to feel good about himself, with a secure sense of self, enjoying good self-esteem and functioning smoothly and harmoniously without undue anxiety and depression— he must experience himself consciously or unconsciously as sur-rounded by the responsiveness of others. The mode of this respon-siveness varies from simple to complex and changes age-appro-priately. Archaic modes are characterized by the need for the ministering physical presence of caregiving others; in maturely rip-ened modes, the needs for selfobject responsiveness are often highly complex and can be met by symbolic representatives supplied by and characteristic of the general culture. In all cases, some responsive selfobject experience is always needed, at least unconsciously. This is true for men, women, and children from birth until death. An ambience of responsiveness is as essential for psychological health as an ambience of a plentiful supply of oxygen is essential for physical health (Wolf, 1980c).

Fragmentation and Symptoms

The person whose self *regresses* from a state of cohesion to one of partial or total loss of structure experiences this as a loss of self-esteem, or as a feeling of emptiness or depression or worthlessness, or anxiety. This change in the structured state of the self has been termed fragmentation. Fragmentation occurs in varying degrees and does not imply complete dissolution of the self. Generally, when we talk about someone fragmenting, we mean a degree of regression associated with symptoms of subjective discomfort. However, frag-mentation is sometimes experienced as the terrifying certainty of imminent death, which signals a process of apparently irreversible dissolution of the self. The experience of a crumbling self is so unpleasant that people will do almost anything to escape the percep-tions brought about by fragmentation.

The term fragmentation unfortunately is often misunderstood. Fragmentation means regression of the self toward lessened cohe-sion, more permeable boundaries, diminished energy and vitality, and disturbed and disharmonious balance. All these take place in degrees of severity and not necessarily equally in each sector of the personality. To be sure, when regression proceeds without limitations beyond control it inevitably leads to the psychological state that we generally understand by the term psychosis. Most fragmentations do not result in psychosis but are characterized by regression of specific aspects of the self and its functioning. Indeed, everyone, at times, experiences some regressive episodes in response to the stressful experiences, specific to our own self structure, to which we all are heir.

Illustration

Let me use a literary depiction from Jean-Paul Sartre's novel *Nausea* to illustrate fragmentation (Sartre, 1938)

Roquentin, the novel's protagonist, who reports his self-experience, uses the symptom of nausea as a label for his disorganized self, his fragmentation. Quite early he tells us the central fact of his existence when he says that he lives alone, entirely alone, and even feels alone when in the midst of happy, reasonable voices (p. 8). Note that aloneness for Sartre does not mean being without people around him, but being without selfobject experiences even in the presence of people. Sartre's description of the experience of inner disorganization that comes with such utter aloneness is unsurpassed. First, there is the sudden awkwardness of bodily movements, the loss of muscular coordination and of sensory preception: Roquentin feels strange, his hand seems changed in the way it picks up a pipe or fork or holds a doorhandle (p. 4). A familiar face suddenly looks unknown, and street noises become suspicious (p. 4). Life has become "jerky, incoherent" (p. 5). It seems that the fragmentation of his self is projected also on to his perception of the world. The self has lost its sense of direction. Roquentin notices being paralyzed, unable to express himself, as though he were full of "lymph and milk" and yet "feeling empty" (p. 5). No longer is it possible to tell "clear, plausible stories" (p. 7). In other words, the world no longer makes sense, meaning has been lost, even the structure or boundaries of the self seem lost when "you plunge into stories without beginning or end" (p. 7). Roquentin is obsessed by the life history of the Marquis de Rollebon, and we soon see that the Marquis's life also seems to have been subject to the kinds of abrupt turns that elude Roquentin's self-understanding: The reports "do not contradict each other, neither do they agree with each other; they do not seem to be about the same person." Lacking is "firmness and consistency" (p. 13), or, as we might paraphrase, cohesion has been lost to fragmentation. In reconstructing the Marquis's life history, Roquentin is trying to make sense of his own history—an effort at self-healing akin to the efforts in psychotherapy to heal through making sense out of the patient's history.

We know that Roquentin is really talking about himself. When he looks into the mirror, his face is just a "gray thing," no longer having sense or direction. In fact, except for the beautiful red hair, he compares his face to a clod of earth or a block of stone; "obviously there are a nose, two eyes, and a mouth, but none of it makes sense, there is not even a human expression" (p. 16).

Sartre even illustrates the causal sequence of the unexpected absence of the needed selfobject, followed by the regression of the self to a state of fragmentation.

Roquentin has gone to the cafe expectantly, but when the waitress informs him that the patronne is out shopping, he feels a disagreeable tingling in his genitals; his vision is fogged by a colored mist (reminiscent of patients telling their therapist that they feel in a fog when they are in a fragmented state). Roquentin sees a whirlpool of lights, smoke, mirrors, and is no longer able to recognize people. He floats, dazed, becomes nauseous, cannot move his head, which feels as though it were elastic and unattached (pp. 18-19). No longer is the nausea within him; he is the one who is within it (p. 20). In other words, his self has lost its boundaries and orientation in space; instead of a meaningfully and cohesively organized set of experiences, that is, a self, it has become an incoherent and disorganized collection of experiences.

Sartre's diagnosis is straight to the point: "In order to exist, [people] also must consort with others" (p. 6). Otherwise they will, like Roquentin, experience a sudden estrangement from themselves in a somato-physiologic manner: the nausea. The sudden loss of inner cohesion is experienced as a sudden senselessness of the world, a strange and disconcerting absurdity. The one place where sense remains, vaguely, for which he strives as the concluding hope of the novel, is the unity and intelligibility of a song—which I would interpret as bringing cognition and affect into a new cohesion, thereby reconstituting the self. As Iris Murdoch (1953) states: "For Roquentin all value lies in the unattainable world of intelligible completeness."

When Sartre demonstrates here his perceptive awareness of the experiences that the vicissitudes of life may heap upon a self, he is by no means an exception among twentieth-century writers. Franz Kafka's *Metamorphosis* vividly depicts the experience of loss of a human self and turning into a nonhuman as a consequence of destructive selfobject experiences (Kohut, 1977, pp. 287–288; Wolf, 1978). Virginia Woolf's *To The Lighthouse*, almost overtly biographical, takes us deeply into the inner lives of the various selfs that constitute the Ramsay (= Stephen, Woolf's family of origin) family; through the character of Lily Briscoe, Woolf illuminates the problems of the creativeness of the self (Wolf & Wolf, 1979). A day in the life of narcissistic personality could be the subtitle of Woolf's *Mrs. Dalloway* (Wolf, 1978). Kohut, like Freud, found much to learn and to inspire him in literature. Shakespeare, Trollope, Kleist, Melville, Thomas Mann, Proust, and O'Neill are among the most important literary influences on Kohut (1977). He sparked a still expanding interest among psychoanalysts to elucidate the insights of writers into the vicissitudes of self experience (Wolf, 1980–1981).

Other Symptomatic Behavior

The subjective experience of a regressing, fragmenting self is so painful in loss of self-esteem and anxiety that emergency measures are instituted to reverse the process. Attempts to boost one's self-esteem often take the form of some sort of self-stimulation; or one provokes or manipulates the environment to supply the needed selfobject experience in order to maintain some structural cohesion to one's self. The resulting behavior often has great social impact and may lead to antagonistic or otherwise counterproductive reverberations. It is annoying for most people to have to listen to a lot of bragging or to witness someone's arrogant attitude, even when one recognizes that such behavior clearly means that someone is suffering and trying to prevent a worse calamity. Much of the irritation of people with each other, the quarrels that tear up marriages, and the misunderstandings that lead to loss of spouse, friend, or job can be traced back to the ups and downs of self-esteem when individuals with fragile selfs try to use others to make themselves feel stronger and more whole.

"Acting out" is a variety of symptomatic behavior. The experience of loss of self that is associated with deep regressions and fragmentations is so painful that individuals will do almost anything to avoid it. From this arises the imperative urge for acting out as a way to ameliorate the fragmented self-experience. Frantic life styles, drug abuse, perversions, and delinquency all serve as desperate measures to hold on to some self-organization and avoid sliding into the fragmented state. Alcohol intoxication and bizarre conduct are often used to distract oneself from the unbearable aspects of fragmentation. Indeed, there are all kinds of excitements that can be used to keep away the feeling of deadness in the self. One can begin to understand from this how some people become compulsive gamblers, others continuously seek the excitement of daredevil activities, and still others become "workaholics" to maintain their sense of selfhood (Kohut & Wolf, 1978).

Transferring the Past into the Present

The vicissitudes of early self experience, when the newly emerging self is at its most vulnerable, force upon the youngster all kinds of distortions to maintain and defend a modicum of unitary and cohesive structure. The self of infancy and childhood may respond to traumatic threats to its cohesion by modifying its structure. For example, in some children the deprivation of needed mirroring selfobject experiences leads to a compensatory intensification, with a resulting overbalancing of the self's pole of ideals. Such selfs are not necessarily pathological, but they will give the personality a cast toward remaining ideal-hungry. In some instances, the idealized pole becomes so dominant that one may speak of the self almost having become identical with the idealized structure. The type of personality that Kohut (1985, pp. 195–202) speaks about as *messianic leaders* has such a self structure, where the self is dominated by its idealizations. Other modifications may be made by splitting the self horizontally to repress some perceptions into inaccessible unconscious regions, or by splitting the self vertically to exclude (to deny or disavow) other perceptions from immediate attention, though these are still accessible to conscious awareness. Another variety of adaptation by alterations in the self is an apparent withdrawal from the selfobject milieu, accompanied by decreasing sensitivity to the surroundings, but compensated by the tension arc of talents and skills becoming the major focus of self awareness. Such a person becomes the typical "organization man" who derives his self-satisfaction from dutifully exercising his skills without too much concern for either mirroring or idealizing needs.

All these changes in the self serve to maintain an optimal cohesion, vigor, and harmony in the face of an inimical selfobject ambience. They are instituted at the cost of both structural and energic impairment that may be so great as to slow or even halt normal development. It is as if a child were clothed in a suit of protective armor whose heaviness forced him to grow into grotesque shapes and drained him of energy. Worse yet, after wearing the armor for some years, the growing body becomes so structurally distorted that the armor can no longer be taken off, even though the dangers against which it protected have passed. For all practical purposes, it is as if the armor has become part of the skin and keeps away not only the archaic dangers, but also the always needed and longed for soft warm human touches. The psychological makeup imposed on a child remains in adulthood, indeed, throughout life.

The clinical manifestation in the adult of this child psychological make-up we call *transference*. In other words, transferences are the fears, the defenses, and the distortions imposed by early traumatic threats to the self that manifest in relations with others in later life when they are no longer appropriate. However, not all transferences are automatically active at all times. Rather, selected transferences are triggered by certain situations or perceptions that remind the individual of the archaic dangers to which he or she was exposed. Thus, transference always has at least two components: the archaic residue of past emergency reactions to danger, which have become chronic character armor, and the repetition in the here-and-now of some perception, that because of its apparent similarity to past experiences of trauma, triggers the archaic pattern in the present.

It is important to remember, however, that not all transference-like phenomena occurring in the therapeutic situation are true transferences, even though they might relate to the therapist. For instance, behavior of the therapist that is grossly deviant from average expectable social discourse—unless understood and *accepted* as necessary for achieving the agreed-upon goal of the therapeutic relationship—will evoke reactions on the part of the patient that are appropriate to the therapist's transgression of social boundaries and are not just a transference of defensive maneuvers from the past. For example, if the therapist is hostile or insulting, the patient will normally and appropriately react with anger. This is not transfer-ence—and it is not transference if the patient reacts angrily to the therapist's silences or other behaviors as hostile or insulting or disrespectful or noxious when compared to average expectable and appropriate social intercourse. On the other hand, with the proper preparation, some patients can learn to accept apparently deviant behavior on part of the therapist, if they understand the need for it in order to achieve certain goals.

An analogy from medical practice comes to mind. Patients usually submit to the most intimate inspection and even painful manipulation by their physician if they understand the necessities demanding such actions. For most patients, however, no matter how well the therapist may try to rationalize the behavior, an attitude of cold detachment that is experienced as an ambience of indifference is not acceptable in either medical or psychotherapeutic practice. Pa-tients may grudgingly learn to put up with it—and in those aspects of medical-surgical practice that do not require the active coopera-tion of the patient, it may not matter much to the success of the attempted procedures—but in psychotherapeutic practice, where the patient's active participation and cooperation is a *sine qua non* for success, it becomes the therapeutic responsibility of the therapist to create an ambience that facilitates rather than hinders the process.

Motivation for Treatment

Relief of psychological pain is the most powerful incentive for seeking treatment. Beyond that, why should a person risk getting hurt again, and why should he or she undergo the painful self-exposure of therapy repeatedly? What is the motivation for subject-ing oneself to the time-consuming, emotionally demanding, and expensive work of psychoanalytic treatment? There is the hope of leading a less painful way of life, the hope to achieve some potential for creative endeavor, and the hope to finally be what one always really could and wanted to be—one's own self expressing itself. But mostly, there is the need for an ambience of being understood, for a self-sustaining selfobject experience that remains always out of reach as long as the archaic defensive patterns get in the way. The search for a healthy wholeness is a search for the sustaining selfobject ambience from which the self can obtain the strength to be whole.

ORIGINS OF SELF PSYCHOLOGY

I shall briefly summarize an overview of the emergence of psychoanalysis and its evolution into self psychology. Psychoanalysis was
the creation of a pioneering genius. Sigmund Freud had both the
strength and the courage to pursue new and generally unacceptable
ideas about human sexuality and aggressiveness by an unsparing self-
examination. In so doing, he created a method for investigating
mental processes, a body of psychological knowledge, and a method
for the treatment of certain psychological illnesses, the so-called
psychoneuroses. Post-Freudian psychoanalysts developed and modified psychoanalysis further, but, in the main, attempted to stay
within the theoretical framework outlined by Freud.

Heinz Kohut, prodded by clinical experiences and enabled by a
courage reminiscent of Freud's, undertook a reexamination and revision of some of the fundamental tenets of psychoanalysis. He clari-
fied the limits of the field by defining it as that part of depth
psychology whose data were obtained with the essential participation
of introspection and empathy (Kohut, 1959). This definition recognizes psychoanalysis as the science of subjectivity, of mental states,
and mental processes. Inevitably, this definition moves the focus of
interest from the psychobiological substrate, the id, and the drives of
classical psychoanalysis, to more purely psychological considerations,
such as the experience of selfhood, its development, and its vicissitudes. The result is a psychoanalytic psychology of the self that is
characterized by a detailed study of the self and its relation to its so-
called selfobjects, that is, to those aspects of the environment that
function to evoke and sustain the varieties of self states and their
manifold manifestations in subjective experience and in behavior.

Self Psychology and Social Issues

Freudian psychoanalysis has taken as its field of investigation
the inner life of the individual. The psychological forces conceptualized are the ones active within the "mental apparatus" and among its
component parts, that is, the id, ego, and superego. Psychoanalysis is
concerned with intra-psychic dynamics. The influences of the environment is not totally ignored in clinical practice, but in theory plays
a secondary role to the *primum mobile*, the instinctual drive. The

objects in the surroundings are used for drive discharge and, in essence, exert their influence by facilitating or frustrating that discharge. Psychic structures such as the superego and ego-identifications arise largely in response to such vicissitudes of drive discharge patterns. Neo-Freudian theorists (Melanie Klein, Fairbairn, Guntrip, Winnicott, Bowlby in Britain; Horney, E. Fromm, H. S. Sullivan, Fromm-Reichmann in the United States) modified the classical theory to give greater recognition to the influence of the needed external object and the surrounding culture. Thus, interpersonal dynamics and object relations have assumed a central position for many contemporary psychoanalysts. However, emphasizing nurture over nature has become the focus of much controversy, more classical Freudians fearing that the really important Freudian discoveries were being watered down or lost by shifting the emphasis from drive to object.

Kohut insisted that self psychology is, like the classical Freudian conceptualizations, an intrapsychic dynamic and not an interpersonal or object-relations theory. Over the two decades of its development, Kohut gradually purged self psychology of instinctual drives and psychic energies—two concepts derived from nineteenth-century natural science—and substituted the phenomenology of conscious and unconscious subjective experience as the stimulus for organizing the psychological structures, foremost the self. Selfobject theory thus became the center of the Kohutian psyche. It is not the reality of the relationship between self and object, but the self's conscious and unconscious experience of that relationship which determines the cohesion, vigor, and harmony of the self.

Clearly, Kohutian self psychology is an individual psychology, not a social psychology. However, I believe that the selfobject concept opens the door to wider issues that traditionally have been the concern of other social scientists. The individual's social role often has a determining effect on the cohesion of his or her self. To put it more precisely, the social role may perform a selfobject function. For example, it is not unusual to observe clinically that some patients with narcissistic personality disorders in a state of self fragmentation achieve a firm and cohesive self structure upon joining an organization. This is accounted for only partially by the recognition they receive (mirroring) or by their ability to idealize individual members in the newly joined organization. Often more decisive is the psychological image of the organization, which can serve as an idealizable selfobject—a source of pride in belonging to it—and may also provide a self-confirming selfobject experience ("I am really somebody now that I am a member"). To give an extreme example, during the height of the post-World War I depression in Germany, the Nazis turned quasi-derelict individuals into efficiently useful ones by putting them into the shiny uniforms of the storm trooper. In other words, self structure was infused with new strength by bolstering it with a strong social identity via selfobject experiences involving the self and an organization functioning as a selfobject. It seems that a social identity can support a crumbling self the way a scaffolding can support a crumbling building.

Some aspects of the relations between leaders and groups can also be illuminated by selfobject theory. Let us assume that groups, like individuals, can form a group self, structured in analogy to individual selfs, with group ambitions and group ideals (Kohut, 1985). We can then understand something about the reciprocal relationship between leaders and followers. Again, a particular crisis may serve as an illustrative case. During the traumatic days after the defeat and evacuation at Dunkirk, the British people—alone, without allies, blockaded into shortages of food and ammunition, the Army in shambles—were in a precarious psychological state verging on defeatism and ineffectiveness. However, a remarkable change occurred when Winston Churchill became Prime Minister. Churchill over many years had built up an image of a strong and fearless person. Through a series of eloquent speeches deriding the Nazis and displaying his own undaunted determination, he was able to imbue his countrymen with his own feelings of power. A *charismatic leader* such as Churchill can, through the hypertrophied pole of ambitions of his bipolar self, repair the defective pole of ambitions of the group self of which he is a part. Analogously, a *messianic leader*, such as Ghandi, can through the hypertrophied pole of ideals of his self instill the needed cohesion into the fragmented group self of his people. The strength and cohesion of the Indian people's group self, which was necessary to suffer triumphantly through a campaign of nonviolence, could not have been mustered without the selfobject experience of that messianic leadership.

Viewing the relations between peoples through the eyes of a self psychologist suggests interpreting these relations as occurring between group selfs. Thus, we can recognize in the jockeying among the great powers—Disarmament, Test Ban, Star Wars, and other negotiations—the fear of each group self to be put into a position of powerlessness. Self psychologists know from their experience with individuals that there is hardly a more frightening situation than the threat of helplessness. Individuals respond to this threat with narcissistic rage—a self's unlimited rage that aims to destroy the origin of the threat to itself. Homicide and suicide are the not uncommon outcomes when there seems to exist no other action to do away with the experience of helplessness. For group selfs, the lessons and their urgency are obvious. One of these appears to be the suggestion that the aim of foreign policy should be the prevention of conditions that favor the arousal of the narcissistic rage of groups, that is, not the weakening but the careful and selective strengthening of potential adversaries.

. 4 .

SELFS AND SELFOBJECTS

As we have discussed, the concept "self" is awkward to define precisely. To be sure, various theorists have defined how they use the term self in their conceptualizations. Such definitions by usage allow one to teach and otherwise communicate what one means. But it is well to keep in mind that such definitions by usage say nothing about the essential nature of a thing. A strict definition has eluded us in self psychology also. However, by observing how self psychology uses the term self, oscillating between describing the transactions of the self and the experiences of the self, I hope to convey the sense of this evolving concept without freezing it into the rigidity of a precise definition. For the moment, that is sufficient for clinical purposes and preserves the fluidity necessary for further theoretical elaborations.

SELF STRUCTURE

The Bipolar Self

Using a spatial metaphor, Kohut describes the self as a bipolar structure (see Chapter 3, page 31). One pole of the self is constituted as a precipitate of mirroring selfobject experiences (discussed later in this chapter, along with idealizing selfobject experiences) and has been designated *the pole of ambitions*. The other pole emerges from idealizing selfobject experiences and has been designated *the pole of values and ideals*. Still speaking metaphorically, *a tension arc* stretches between these poles because the two poles push/pull the self in different directions. Along this tension arc are arrayed the inborn talents and acquired skills.

A Life Plan

At the time when an individual's self first comes into being as a singular and unique specific cohesive structure, the whole configuration of poles and tension arc being laid down is the core of this *nuclear self*. This unique core configuration gives the self an idiosyncratic and specific direction that in its lifelong unfolding can be called a *life plan* for the self. A person who lives in harmony with the self's life plan enjoys a sense of fulfilment. A person who deviates in significant aspects from the self's life plan suffers the chronic discontent that comes with feeling unfulfilled. The French artist Paul Gauguin did not find fulfillment until he abandoned a successful commercial career to become a painter. I have analyzed an artist with a similar psychological history. He had been a very successful executive in a business that made only sporadic and mainly noncreative use of his artistic talents. In spite of ample recognition and financial rewards, he continually suffered a feeling of dissatisfaction, which was relieved only when he finally abandoned his business career to become a full-time artist.

The Balanced Self

When the constituent parts of the self, that is, the two poles as well as the arc of talents and skills, are all present in roughly equal strength, we can speak of a harmoniously balanced self. Often, however, the constituents are weighted unequally. A predominant pole of ambitions is found in charismatic people, whereas a predominant pole of ideals is characteristic for messianic personalities. The bland personality of the "organization man" is characteristic for a self with an overmastering tension arc that dominates at the expense of the two poles.

Some of the leading functionaries of the Nazi party machinery were such organization men, who would superficially strike one as being rather ordinary individuals. They were often good family men, neither outstandingly ambitious for personal gain, nor especially fervent in pursuit of their values. Indeed, they seemed often blandly uninteresting, and the unspeakable evils they committed on a massive scale appear incongruous with the generally quite normal life they led privately. If there was an outstanding quality that they had in common it was, perhaps, their unquestioning dedication and commitment to the organizations of which they were a part and whose aims they adopted totally as their own. The organizer of the Holocaust, Adolf Eichmann, seems a good example of this type of person with an imbalanced self structure: impoverished at the poles of ambition and ideals with a relatively hypertrophied arc of talents and skills.

The Empty Self

Chronic deprivation of self-organizing selfobject experiences leave the self relatively empty of the structured complexity and energic vitality of selfs that grew up in richly responsive environments. Clinically, these people often suffer from a low-grade chronic depressive mood with feelings of emptiness and lack of zest.

The Selfobject

It is not quite as difficult to define the term *selfobject*, although it is much more frequently misunderstood than the term *self*. The most frequent misunderstanding is to think of the selfobject as a person. To be sure, quite frequently the selfobject function is performed by a person, but it is important to remember that the selfobject is the function, not the person.

Referring to a selfobject as if it were a person, that is, an object, would be correct, if imprecise, only from the point of view of the outside observer. It is more in keeping with the clinical basis of self psychology to think about selfobjects from the point of view of the self, that is, as a selfobject *experience*. To be sure, most of the earliest selfobject experiences are experiences brought about by persons, that is, mainly by the earliest caregivers. Thus, it has become convenient to talk about objects having selfobject functions, and it would be awkward to constantly remind the listener or reader that one really means the *experiences* evoked by these objects. Any experience that functions to evoke the structured self (which manifests as an experience of selfhood) or to maintain the continuity of such selfhood is properly designated as a selfobject experience.

Selfobject experiences can be the function not only of objects, but also of symbols or ideas representing objects. Like other selfobject experiences, they serve by performing the specific function of providing a self-evoking and self-sustaining experience to the potential and to the emerged self. Strictly speaking, therefore, selfobjects are neither selfs nor objects, but the *subjective* aspect of a function performed by a relationship. As such, the selfobject relationship refers to an *intrapsychic* experience and does not describe the interpersonal relationship between the self and other objects. It denotes the subjective experience of imagoes that are needed for the sustenance of the self. Thus the hermit who has withdrawn into the desert is not necessarily suffering from selfobject deprivation because of his apparent aloneness. Indeed, such isolation seems to allow some specially gifted people to experience their relationship to religious ideas and figures with an intensity that rivals the most intimate personal selfobject responsiveness.

The ministration of a parent or caretaker will evoke in a child a selfobject experience that leads to the age-appropriate structuring into an organization that we call the self. For instance, a mother, in addressing and caring for and responding to her child, creates for the child a selfobject experience that has a structuring effect on the child's potentials for self-organization so that a self is evoked and maintained. This emerging self, when it achieves a degree of cohesion, is experienced by the child as a sense of selfhood and is accompanied by self-esteem and an experience of well-being. Experiencing the self-evoking and self-maintaining selfobject function is needed by selfs as long as a person lives. Thus a healthy mature self also needs a constant supply of selfobject experiences, but the *form* of these will have undergone a development. For example, an adult might no longer need the extent of physical touching and holding that a child requires, but may get her selfobject experience from reading a novel, or from viewing a particularly moving composition in a painting, or from hearing a certain piece of music that is in tune with her current selfobject needs. Many other such symbolic selfobject experiences replace for the adult the more concrete selfobject experiences needed in infancy and childhood. Religious experiences, group experiences, scientific and philosophic insights, and the like, can be counted among the variety of selfobject experiences that function to maintain selfhood in adulthood.

Because the self-sustaining function of selfobject experiences is needed for life, and because the form of these experiences changes age-appropriately, we can talk about a developmental line of selfobject relations or, more precisely, of selfobject experiences (Wolf, 1980c). In a somewhat schematic way, the selfobject needs can be outlined as follows: (1) A neonate needs a self-evoking experience with a real-life person who, by providing certain tuned-in responses, functions as a selfobject for that neonate: (2) an adolescent needs a self-sustaining experience with real objects or with symbols, such as provided by the adolescent subculture in the form of speech, clothes, music, idols, and so forth, which by their availability function as selfobjects for that particular adolescent. (3) An adult needs a self-sustaining experience with real objects or with symbols, such as provided by art, literature, music, religion, ideas, which by their availability function as selfobjects for that particular adult. For example, an adult might find himself in a rather fragile self-state after a draining experience and then, perhaps, find a self-sustaining selfobject experience by listening to a late Beethoven quartet or a Bach cantata. In this particular experience, he might find himself relating to a nonverbal presence that served to mirror and soothe, whereas, at other times, he might find himself enhanced by relating to an idealized grandeur. These experiences are only partly conscious, but their effect on the self is powerfully strengthening. Other adults might find similar self-sustaining experiences by looking at a painting, reading a novel, seeing a play, going to church, saluting the flag, and so on. It is the subjective aspect of a relationship to an unconscious object mediated by a symbolic presence that becomes effective by providing a selfobject function.

SELFOBJECT EXPERIENCES

Intrapsychic versus Interpersonal

The presence of the selfobject, when it is functioning appropriately, evokes and maintains the self and its concomitant sense of selfhood. This is an intrapsychic event and is subjectively experienced. Selfobject relations, or more precisely, selfobject experiences, are the proper topic for psychoanalytic investigation. Selfobject experiences are not objectively observable from the outside, so to speak. They are not events in an interpersonal context and are not part of social psychology. It is an error to talk about selfobject relations either as object relations or as interpersonal relations. The interpersonal relations between persons may give rise to selfobject experiences and, inferentially, one may guess at the selfobject experiences that accompany certain relations between persons. Direct access to the selfobject experience is only by introspection and empathy.

Outlining Selfobject Needs

To maintain its cohesion, its vigor, and its balance, the healthy self needs to be embedded in a milieu that is experienced as constantly supplying a self-sustaining selfobject ambience. Five types of selfobject need will be differentiated here in schematized outline:

1. *Mirroring needs*: a need to feel affirmed, confirmed, recognized; to be feeling accepted and appreciated, especially when able to show oneself.
2. *Idealizing needs*: a need to experience oneself as being part of an admired and respected selfobject; needing the opportunity to be accepted by and merge into a stable, calm, nonanxious, powerful, wise, protective, selfobject that possesses the qualitites the subject lacks.
3. *Alterego needs*: a need to experience an essential alikeness with the selfobject.
4. *Adversarial needs*: a need to experience the selfobject as a benignly opposing force who continues to be supportive and responsive while allowing or even encouraging one to be in active opposition and thus confirming an at least partial autonomy; the need for the availability of a selfobject experience of assertive and adversarial confrontation *vis-à-vis* the selfobject without the loss of self-sustaining responsiveness from that selfobject.
5. *Merger needs*:
a.   extension of self: a primitive form of the mirroring need that finds confirmation of self only in the experience of being totally one with the mirroring selfobject.
b.   with idealized selfobject: an intensification of the idealizing need that requires being totally one with the idealized selfobject.
6. *Efficacy needs*: a need to experience that one has an impact on the selfobject and is able to evoke needed selfobject experiences.

Infantile versus Mature Selfobject Needs

Mirroring, idealizing, alterego, efficacy and adversarial selfobject needs are present at all ages. *Age-appropriate* selfobject needs are the normally required selfobject experiences that fit the age-dependent requirements to sustain self cohesion. In the infant, archaic selfobject needs are age-appropriate. In the adult, the age-appropriately modified needs are often referred to as mature selfobject needs. The belated manifestations of relatively archaic modes at a later age is evidence for disturbed development and may be psychopathological.

Infantile selfobject needs are the normal and appropriate demands for the normally required selfobject experiences of early childhood. These archaic types of selfobject experience may still be indispensable in later life, either temporarily during periods of stress, or, chronically in the disorders of the self.

Developmental Phases

Archaic Infantile Phase

Merger. Neonates and small infants presumably experience themselves before self/object differentiation as if in a limitless merger with the world. Another way of putting this is to say that the infant in this blissful state expands his self-experience to include the whole surround. It is well to keep in mind, however, that these are anthropomorphic and metaphorical descriptions of the infant's presumed experience and that they do not assume much of a thinking and imagining capacity on the part of the baby. Rather, they refer to inferred experiential states. Even after self/object differentiation and the emergence, at least transiently, of a sense of selfhood and a structured self, there is easy and nonpathological oscillation between states of merger and states of nonmerger. At a later age, such merger states would be indicative of regression and, possibly, pathology.[1]

1.The presumed expansion of the infant's self-experience to include his whole world with himself at the center has been termed, I believe misleadingly, as "infantile grandiosity." But the infant's experience is a grandoise self-conception only in the judgment of the observer; the infant is incapable of judging or conceptualizing, and the term grandiosity does not fit well what is in essence an experience of blissful well-being.

Mirroring. The infant requires mirroring activity by its self-objects because such mirroring experiences are needed to evoke the self structure and its concomitant experience of selfhood. The need for mirroring selfobject experiences remains throughout life.

Idealizing. The need during infancy for the availability of idealizable selfobjects to provide idealizing selfobject experiences for the evocation and sustenance of self structure is equal to the need for mirroring selfobject experiences. Both types of experiences are needed throughout life to evoke and sustain the sense of self.

Alter-ego or Twinship. The need to experience the essential likeness of the selfobject and to be strengthened by its quietly sustaining presence are probably present already during infancy, though we can state with certainty only that needed alter-ego selfobject experiences occur from about the oedipal phase onward.

Adversarial and Efficacy. These needs seem to appear first around the time of emergence of a cohesive self during the second year of life. They remain needed throughout life.

Oedipal Phase

Mirroring, idealizing, adversarial, efficacy and alter-ego selfobject experiences are required during the oedipal period of infantile sexuality in order for the developing self to form adequate gender identity and to prevent the kind of distortions in self structure that leave a disposition for the later outbreak of psychoneurosis in adulthood.

In outline, the requirements are as follows: (1) *Boy*: nonseductive confirmation of autonomy and maleness by mother; acceptance of his idealizing needs. Nonaggressive acceptance of adversarial and alter-ego needs by father. (2) *Girl*: nonseductive confirmation of autonomy, and femaleness by father; acceptance of her idealizing needs. Nonaggressive acceptance of alter-ego and adversarial needs by mother.

Latency Phase

In addition to the always-needed mirroring and idealizing experiences, one observes especially during latency, but also to some extent throughout life, that selfobjects are needed as models to imitate and to provide the experience of likeness. These alter-ego experiences are prominent in the development of skills. They open an avenue for learning from peers and from parents as models.

Prepubertal Phase

During the prepubertal years, a gradual expansion of the various modes of selfobject experiences takes place—with a shift away from the early caretakers as the provider of the selfobject function toward teachers, friends, and, most importantly, symbolic substitutes for the selfobject person. The selfobject modes are becoming more diffuse and less personal.

Adolescent and Young Adult Phase

The process begun in the prepubertal phase becomes more encompassing and deeper during adolescence. Cognitive development leads to a recognition of parental defects, with the inevitable outcome of a rapid de-idealization of the early idealized selfobjects. Because the self cannot exist in the selfobject vacuum caused by the de-idealization of parental imagoes, but only in relationship to responsive selfobjects, the adolescent turns to the peer group, to the adolescent subculture and its idols, and to the heroes of cultural history for the needed selfobject sustenance. The availability of the peer group to substitute for parents as idealized selfobjects can be crucial for the maintenance of psychological health. The availability of cultural selfobjects for idealization, for example, heroes of history, art, religion, and ideas, allows for the reconstruction of values and integration into the general culture.

During the adolescent developmental process the idealized parental imago is normally replaced, at least temporarily, by idealized imagoes from the adolescent's subculture. These change with what is fashionable in the subculture. Eventually the adolescent creates his or her own idealized set of values that will also contain aspects of the parental ideals and will be partially in harmony with the general culture, partially critical of the old values and traditions.

These developmental processes require that the adolescent have a period in life where little is required for him or her to contribute to the family or the larger social unit until later in development. Such a moratorium, as Erikson has termed it, is experienced by the adolescent with much ambivalence. While it is pleasant to have the time, the leisure, the funds, and the fun, it is humiliating to have no scope for taking real responsibility. The challenge to be somebody now rather than in the indefinite future is irresistible for many young people and leads to much turmoil. Some adolescents substitute an alter-ego selfobject experience for the normally occurring idealization of the peer-group idols. This can lead to a dangerous turn of events because the alter-ego will be chosen in the likeness of the adolescent's self and thus confirms the deficiencies and faults of the latter, rather than enriching it with new possibilities.

Marital Phase

Spouses are used by each other for a variety of selfobject functions. Intimacy facilitates controlled regression to primitive merger without fear of irreversibly losing the autonomy of the self. Expansion of self boundaries to include the spouse allows participation in the self-sustaining selfobject experience of the other as if it were the self. On the other hand, frustrations and disappointments in the expected and needed selfobject experiences threaten the cohesion of the self and may lead to behaviors that threaten the marriage.

Parenthood Phase

Ideally, parents have sufficiently solid and cohesive selfs to facilitate sufficient flexibility and fluidity as needed by their offspring. Fluidity of self boundaries also makes it possible to include children as selfobjects or to let them separate autonomously, as needed by both children and parents. Weissman and Cohen (1985) have recently demonstrated that the *parenting alliance* is a needed self–selfobject relationship vital to the evolving parenthood experience and other adult tasks.

Middle-age Phase

Middle age is a time for self-evaluation. Therefore, the individual needs selfobjects that will accept the self's reassessment of itself and the readjustment of its goals (social, vocational, career, family) in accord with the self's action plan expressed in its life curve. Significant deviation from that plan results in an experience of nonfulfilment that may eventuate in a so-called midlife crisis.

Old-age Phase

Old age is characterized by the need to idealize the community and to be confirmed as an especially valuable guide and model for the community's ideals.

Efficacy Experiences

The selfobject experiences discussed so far have mostly had in common that they referred to the self as the recipient of some action of the selfobject. Even when these actions of the selfobject were somehow evoked by the self having made its needs known, these selfobject experiences focused primarily on the selfobject as the actor and the self as acted upon. I would like to examine now another group of phenomena that proceed in the opposite direction, that is, phenomena characterized by the self as the actor and the selfobject as the acted-upon. Because the essence of these phenomena is the self's experience of being an effective agent in influencing the object, one might call these phenomena efficacy experiences. It seems likely that such efficacy experiences are as important for the evocation of the sense of self as the previously discussed selfobject experiences, and, therefore, one may also speak of the self's efficacy needs.

In 1905, Freud had mentioned an apparatus for obtaining mastery (1905b, p. 159) and an instinct of mastery (1905b, p. 193). Elaborating in 1913 he wrote, "Activity is supplied by the common instinct of mastery, which we call sadism when we find it in the service of the sexual function" (1913b, p. 322) and "Indeed it is at bottom a sublimated off-shoot of the instinct of mastery exalted into something intellectual, and its repudiation in the form of doubt plays a large part in the picture of obsessive neurosis." (1913b, p. 324) And again, in 1920, in the discussion of the *fort-da* game he speculated, "These efforts might be put down to an instinct for mastery that was acting independently of whether the memory was in itself pleasurable or not." (1920a, p. 16) However, he did not pursue this line of investigation. Angyal (1941), in a similar vein, discussed a "trend to autonomy," which was mentioned by Hendrick (1943, p. 315) when he elaborated on what he chose to call an instinct to master. He characterized it as a fundamental drive of human beings to control the environment and associated it with a specific pleasure experience that he termed work pleasure. Hendrick (1942) referred here to "an inborn drive to do and to learn how to do. This instinct appears to determine more of the behavior of the child during the first two years than even the need for sensual pleasure" (p. 40). However, Hendrick's view received little acceptance.

Research on Infants

Recent data reported from research on infants strongly suggest a reexamination of the relevance for psychoanalytic theories of structure formation of the mutual interaction between infants and mothers. White (1959) studied what he called the "concept of competence" based on infant observations. He concluded that activities in the ultimate service of competence must therefore be conceived to be motivated in their own right, proposed that this motivation be designated "effectance," and characterized the experience produced as a feeling of "efficacy" (p. 329).

Furthermore, Lichtenberg has shown that more recent researches in infant development are suggestive of the role of efficacy pleasure in the consolidation of self experience (Lichtenberg, 1983, 1988).[2]

> In a classic example demonstrating infant's pleasure in their own efficacy four-month-old infants were exposed to five seconds of multicolored bursts of light (Papousek, 1975). "They oriented themselves toward the stimulation with interest, and then, typical of responses to unvaried stimuli, their orientation diminished after repetition. The experiment was arranged so that when the infants in the course of their movements rotated their head 30 degrees to a predetermined side three times successively within a time interval, the light display was switched on. As soon as the infants turned on the light presentation by their own head movements, their behavior changed dramatically. Their orientation reactions increased in intensity, and they continuously made all kinds of movement to try to switch on the visual

2. Various infant researchers have used different terms in reporting on the phenomena here discussed. Efficiency, competence pleasure, efficacy pleasure, and effectance pleasure are among these (cf. White, 1959; Papousek, 1975; Broucek, 1979; and Sander, 1983).

stimulation again. To this point, the experiment would seem to be simply a proof of classical conditioning of a stimulus-response. But the Papouseks then made a significant observation. They found that the infants, after a few successes, may leave their head turned 90 degrees even though the lights were to be seen in the midline. Furthermore, the infants did not seem to be watching. Nonetheless, they continued to turn on the display and responded to their success with smiles and happy bubbling." (Lichtenberg, 1988)

Other infant researchers also observed that when infants have contingent control over events in the external world they begin to smile. Broucek (1979, p. 312) believes the source of pleasure does not lie in problem solving alone but from those experiences in which the infant's activity is the cause of the result. He concludes that awareness of being the cause and the sense of efficacy and pleasure associated with it are the foundation of self feeling. Lichtenberg has identified the sense of achieving physiological regulation due to a satisfactory match between caregiver ministrations and the infant's awareness of need as a foundation of self feeling. Furthermore, he indicates that achieving intimacy in attachment and affiliation to be another foundation of self feeling (Lichtenberg, 1988). The characteristic patterns of mutual influence of mother and infant come to be recognized and expected by the infant (Bebee & Lachmann, 1988; Stern, 1974). Thus, there exists now a body of data that illuminates structure formation in infancy and, by extension, may also illuminate the restoration of structure in psychoanalytic treatment.

The Experience of Efficacy in Psychoanalytic Treatment

From the awareness of having an initiating and causal role in bringing about states of attachment and intimacy, the infant acquires an *experience of efficacy* that—in addition to the responsive selfobject experiences—becomes an essential aspect of the cohesive self-experience. It is as if the infant were able to say to himself (with apologies to René Descartes): I can elicit a response, therefore I am somebody. The regression facilitated during the analysis of adults opens the way to reexperiencing on an archaic level the pleasurable experience of efficacy and the painful self-destroying experience of the loss of efficacy. (See also discussion of transference restoration, Chapter 9, pp. 114–115.)

SUMMARY

There has been a subtle but discernable shift in our major focus toward the selfobject rather than the self as our center of conceptual gravity. This shift has come about for a number of reasons. One is the inescapable recognition that we never observe selfs in a vacuum, so to speak, but only within a framework of a matrix of selfobject experiences provided by the functioning of selfobjects. The self resists precise definition. The selfobject concept, however, difficult though it is to comprehend at first, can be defined fairly precisely in terms of the self: Selfobjects are those experiences that evoke, maintain, and give cohesion to the self. Objects, of course, perform many psychological functions for the person—for example, they may give sexual pleasure, they may feed or support in a variety of ways, they may teach skills, protect, and so on. Some of these interpersonal functions that objects perform in a variety of ways may secondarily, because of the pleasure and success they give to the self, be supportive for the self without being necessary for the integrity of the self's structure. These interpersonal functions are to be distinguished from those selfobject functions that as selfobject experiences are sustaining the self.

Let me illustrate this most important distinction by recalling, for example, a common vicissitude of the student-teacher relationship. Let's say a student contracts with a teacher in order to study music. In the beginning, the student uses the teacher to learn some musical skill. The relationship is an interpersonal one with an interpersonal function. Generally, after a few weeks, if there are disappointments, the relationship can be broken off or the teacher exchanged for another without any psychological pain of any consequence to either party. But sometimes, perhaps because of some special need of one or the other—not necessarily an abnormal need—the relationship changes: Now, any disruption is experienced by one or both as a significant psychological trauma—and may even lead to a psychotic break if the relationship is broken off. One recognizes that an intense reaction has developed and is jeopardizing the relationship. Some archaic selfobject need has become mobilized and requires a specific selfobject experience in order to maintain the cohesion of the self. Because it manifests in the present as a revival of an archaic need, we call this phenomenon a *selfobject transfer-*

ence: The self of one or both of the participants has become dependent on the other for the needed selfobject support to its self. What had been an interpersonal relationship dedicated to the acquisition of skills has been superseded by a selfobject experience functioning to maintain the structure and cohesion of the self.

.5.

SELFOBJECT RELATIONS DISORDERS: DISORDERS OF THE SELF

DEFINITION

Significant failure to achieve cohesion, vigor, or harmony of the self may be said to constitute a state of self disorder. Speaking etiologically, that means a *selfobject relations disorder* or, more precisely, a disorder due to faulty selfobject experiences.

ETIOLOGY

Throughout the course of life, the self is vulnerable to the absence, insufficiency, or inappropriateness of selfobject experiences. This vulnerability is greatest during the formative years, but injuries to the self can occur at any age. At major developmental turning points, such as the oedipal phase, early adolescence, marriage, parenthood, mid-life, or upon entering old age—the so-called *life crises*—there appears to be a heightened vulnerability of the self to being injured by inappropriate selfobject experiences.

Faulty interaction between the child and his or her caregivers, especially during the early years when the self first emerges, is experienced by the nascent self[1] as dangerous or even injurious selfobject responsiveness. The resulting traumatic selfobject experiences lead to a diffusely damaged self or to a self that is seriously damaged in one or the other of its constituents. The disorders of the

---

1. Clearly, it is imprecise and, at worst, incorrect to speak about the self as if it were an existential agent. I should be speaking about a person whose self's strengths or weaknesses lead to experiences of agency. Kohut said that the self is a center of initiative. This shortened definition of agency is less awkward than spelling out the distinction between self and person each time.

self are, by and large, but not exclusively, the consequence of miscarriages in the normal development of the self. It is difficult to state precisely the age at which the baby or small child may be said to have acquired a self. To begin with, it seems safe to assume that, strictly speaking, the neonate is still without a self. The new-born infant arrives physiologically pre-adapted for a specific physical environment—the presence of oxygen, of food, of a certain range of temperature—outside of which he or she cannot survive. Similarly, psychological survival requires a specific psychological environment—the presence of responsive–empathic selfobjects providing needed selfobject experiences. These needed experiences give firmness and cohesion to the child's fragile self. A list of needed experiences would include at least four different kinds of responses from his selfobject environment.

Mirroring Selfobject Experiences. These provide confirmation for the child's innate sense of vigor, greatness (wonderfulness), and perfection.

A nine-year-old was playing ball with some other children when he hit the ball through the basement window of a neighbor's house, breaking it. The boy's mother was able to respond in a self-sustaining manner by appreciating with a "Wow, that must have been quite a well-hit ball," but also by recognizing that her son was old enough to take some responsibility for his actions: She told him that he would have to help pay for the damage out of his allowance. This is an example of a mirroring selfobject experience.

When the boy's father heard about this in the evening, he angrily threatened that the boy would not get the new bat he'd been promised if anything like this happened again. This is an example of a faulty selfobject experience.

Idealized Selfobject Experiences. These are available to the child as emanating from images of calmness, infallibility, and omnipotence, with which the child can merge.

Jackie, a talented teenager, had been given the lead role in a school play. The parents proudly attended the play and greatly enjoyed it. This was a positive mirroring experience for the girl. Afterward, at a get-together of parents and cast members, Jackie's father inappropriately pulled out a hip flask and noisily toasted his daughter. Under the circumstances, this was totally unacceptable behavior, and Jackie felt terribly ashamed of her father's *faux pas*. This was a faulty idealizing selfobject experience.

Alter-ego Selfobject Experiences. These are needed to become models and provide experiences of likeness that sustain the self and that stimulate the potential for learning.

Adversarial Selfobject Experiences. These are needed for healthy assertiveness *vis-à-vis* the caregiver without fear of impairing the selfobject relationship (cf. Wolf, 1976a).

John wanted to borrow the family car to take some friends to a rock concert. However, his parents strongly disapproved of one particular friend, Harry, because he was known to be involved with drugs. John believed that he could handle Harry, but the parents insisted that John would not get the car unless he first promised not to let Harry ride with him. John became very angry, but he eventually accepted his parents conditions under protest as the price for getting the car and maintaining a good relationship with them. This was an adversarial selfobject experience for parents and child both.

Faulty interactions—more precisely, psychologically traumatic selfobject experiences—between a child and his or her caregivers result in a damaged self that predisposes the individual to a later outbreak of a disorder of the self. Depending on the nature of the damage, therefore, adult selfs exist in varying degrees of *cohesion*, have various levels of *vigor*, and are balanced in varying degrees of *harmony*.

CLASSIFICATION

The Selfobject Relations Disorders can be subdivided usefully into a number of groups according to the nature of the damage to the self.

Psychoses. If the damage to the self is relatively permanent, and the defect is not covered over by defenses, then the resulting syndrome is like those that are traditionally referred to as the psychoses.

Constitutional factors combine with the effects of deficient mirroring to produce the noncohesive psychopathology of schizophrenia. In another category, inherent organic factors combine with the psychological depletion resulting from lack of joyful selfobject responses to leave a predisposition toward empty depression. The absence of structure-building experiences, which normally attend the merger with calm idealized selfobjects, is likely to result in insufficient self-soothing structures or self-supportive structures and, therefore, predisposes the individual to mania or guilt depression.

Borderline States. These are characterized by similar, relatively permanent injuries to the self, except that the damage is covered by complex defenses. A borderline self may protect its fragile structure against further serious damage from both the rough-and-tumble and the intimacy of social intercouse (1) by using schizoid mechanisms to keep involvement shallow, or (2) by using paranoid mechanisms to surround itself with an aura of hostility and suspicion that will keep noxious selfobjects at bay.

Though there have been many attempts to specify criteria for the psychopathology and diagnosis of borderline states, it seems evident that none of them are really satisfactory. In practice, the word *borderline* has become a wastebasket term signifying severe pathology in patients who present particularly difficult treatment problems characterized by intense affect reactions and frequently by acting out. Beyond this generalized statement, no specific constellation of symptoms can be described that would allow a reliable diagnosis of borderline state. Conceptually, Kohut and I have characterized the psychopathology of borderline states as a permanent or protracted break-up, enfeeblement, or functional chaos of the nuclear self—the experiential and behavioral manifestations of which, in contrast to the psychoses, are covered by complex defenses (Kohut & Wolf, 1978, p. 415). How are these conditions to be diagnosed, then, when no reliable symptom picture can be drawn? In accord with our dynamic formulation and with our conceptualization of the therapeutic process, I would think it generally almost impossible to diagnose a borderline condition without having some information about how the therapeutic process unfolded with that particular patient. In other words, reliable diagnosis is possible only on the basis of observing the transference during a trial of therapy or analysis.

When affective reactions of the patient to the therapist's inevitable faulty responses (inevitably nonattuned responses) are so severe and associated with acting out that is not acceptable to the therapist (and often also not acceptable to the patient), then we can usually label the patient as borderline.

At the present time, therefore, we have to classify the borderline states as a disorder of the self but not a narcissistic personality disorder nor a narcissistic behavior disorder; in other words, as a separate diagnostic category. With continued progress in theory and treating self disorders I would hope that eventually the category borderline would dissolve into a small group who are psychotic and a much larger group whom we can understand and treat as narcissistic behavior disorders. At the present time we are most handicapped by our empathic inabilities, that is, by our not yet understanding enough about the borderline experience to really become attuned to such patients.

Narcissistic Behavior Disorders. Less severe and more temporary damage to the self is found in the narcissistic behavior disorders. Characteristically, these persons attempt to shore up their crumbling self-esteem through perverse, delinquent, or addictive behavior.

Narcissistic Personality Disorders. In the narcissistic personality disorders, we find even less severely damaged selfs. Here the injured state of the self is experienced directly in the form of subjective symptomatology, such as hypochondria, depression, hypersensitivity to slights, lack of zest, inability to concentrate on tasks, irritability, insomnia, and so forth.

Psychoneuroses. The psychoneuroses proper are a special variant of the narcissistic personality disorders, and are the result of faulty selfobject experiences with oedipal selfobjects during the oedipal phase. They are characterized by neurotic symptoms, such as the symptoms of anxiety, depression, or phobia; or conversions, such as paralysis, paresis, paresthesias, anesthesias, or certain other somatic phenomena; or obsessive thinking or compulsive behavior. When overt sexual feelings and desires manifest during the treatment of psychoneurotic syndromes, it is sometimes difficult to distinguish the mobilization of oedipal sexual transferences from the sexualization of needed selfobject experiences.

PSYCHOPATHOLOGY (SELF STATES)

A chronically faulty selfobject environment, rather than single traumatic events, causes the developmental failures that leave the child vulnerable, with specific constellations of damage to the self. Certain characteristic types of self pathology stand out, although they are usually found in mixtures rather than in pure culture.

Understimulated Selfs. Prolonged lack of stimulating responsiveness from the selfobjects of childhood results in understimulated selfs. Such people lack vitality and experience themselves as boring. In order to ward off painful feelings of deadness, they need to create a pseudo-excitement by the use of any available stimulus. Depending on the developmental phase, one may see head-banging among toddlers, compulsive masturbation in children, and daredevil activities in adolescents and adults. Adults, of course, can be quite inventive in producing innumerable kinds of self-stimulating behavior. As examples may serve such diverse activities as deviant sexuality, drug and alcohol abuse, and frenzied life styles in business or in social spheres. Even such splendid exercises as jogging or running can be transformed into pathological excesses by a self's need for stimulation to maintain its cohesion. The "highs" that can be experienced during these self-stimulating exertions are familiar to all of us and are a reminder of the extraordinary sense of well-being enjoyed by a really cohesive self. On the other hand, in a damaged self, because the joy provided by healthy functioning of the total self is unavailable, the ubiquitous empty depression is kept at bay by creating pleasurably stimulating sensations in parts of the body or mind.

A 53-year-old accountant came into treatment because of moderate chronic depression and anxiety, which made his daily life a miserable experience, though he was able to perform his work well. He was constantly concerned that he was not really fully accepted by his partners; in fact, he felt that he did not really belong anywhere. He exuded a general aura of pessimism and negativism. There was no trace of enthusiasm for anything—either people or objects. Occasionally he would engage his wife in bitter discussions expounding his black view of the world, and the arguments that developed could evoke a kind of pseudo-excitement in him. He had been born in Western Europe to moderately well-off parents. His father was a grocer, his mother helped in the store, and their two children were cared for by a series of maids. The vicissitudes of war caused the patient's separation from his parents at age seven, and subsequently he grew up in a series of foster homes in America. It is not clear why he was unable to make any lasting human relationships in any of these homes, but a chronic bed-wetting problem may have been an important factor. During treatment it became apparent, from both the reconstruction of his history as well as from manifestations in the transference, that he had no expectation of any real interest in him from anybody. Yet equally apparent was his need for recognition and confirmation of his worth by his coworkers and, especially, from me. His understimulated self manifested as a chronic depression.

Fragmented Selfs. Lack of integrating responses to the emerging infantile self predispose the individual to states of partial fragmentation. Such people react to narcissistic injuries with a disturbed sense of the continuity of their self or the smoothness of its functioning. Characteristically, they are anxious, hypochondriacal, and awkward and clumsy in posture, gait, or speech.

A thirty-five-year-old research chemist was unhappy with his professional career because of lack of advancement, though he had been well trained by an Ivy League University. His first marriage had ended in divorce when his wife, tired of his obsessive–compulsive nagging, ran off with a college boyfriend. The patient suffered greatly from a number of minor illnesses that assumed life-threatening proportions in his mind. His awkward posture and clumsy movements, as well as his chronically morose anxiety, had caused him to be ridiculed by his college classmates, resulting in a general feeling of mortified alienation. He was the only child of two chronically sick, elderly parents who, though well-meaning, were quite unable to adequately respond to their youngster. They were at once overprotective, impatient, and authoritarian. From this confusing milieu he withdrew into a rich fantasy life, and he compensated himself with the deserved recognition he received for his outstanding intellectual achievements at school. But underneath this compensating structure he remained in a partially fragmented state. In treatment he responded well to the integrating effect provided by a stable and accepting therapeutic ambience.

Overstimulated Selfs. Excessive or inappropriate selfobject responses may lead to an overstimulated state of the self. These people are fearful of the tension induced by being flooded with fantasies of their own greatness or excited fantasies about the greatness of others. As a consequence, these persons will be shy or lack the normal capacity for enthusiastically pursuing a goal.

Overburdened Selfs. Overburdened selfs did not have the opportunity to merge with the calmness of an omnipotent selfobject. Therefore, such individuals lack the self-soothing structures that protect the normal individual from being traumatized by the spreading of his or her emotions. Even gentle stimuli cause painful excitement, and the world is experienced as hostile and dangerous. Somatic hyperirritability and migraines have been observed.

A woman in her early thirties had married a widower with three teenage children. The children's mother had died following a sudden overwhelming illness. The patient's father had been a somewhat sociopathic man whose acting out behavior had led to his premature sudden death when his daughter was not yet in her teens. The patient's mother had been an overly anxious woman, more concerned with the neighbors' good opinion of her than with the traumatic shock to her daughter caused by the father's untimely and disreputable demise. In fact, the mother accused the little girl of being very much like her father, and by a kind of loose association she was burdened with some responsibility for her father's sins. Or so at least it seemed to her. During treatment, she often experienced even gentle questions as assaultive, and at times she would think the whole psychoanalytic situation was inimical. At such times, or when extra-analytical demands on her were especially heavy, she might suffer attacks of migraine headache.

CHARACTEROLOGY (BEHAVIORAL PATTERNS)

So far I have discussed psychopathology, that is, the different types of pathological states of the self that we have learned to distinguish. I come now to different types of behavioral patterns that are characteristic of all disorders of the self, including the narcissistic personality disorders. Although narcissistic behavior disorders refer specifically to prominent and acute acting-out behavior, such as delinquency, addiction, and perversion, narcissistic personality disorders also express aspects of their psychopathology in their behavior and, thus, also give rise to characteristic chronic behavioral patterns.

Mirror Hungry Personality. Mirror hungry personalities are impelled to display themselves to evoke the attention of others, who through their admiring responses will perhaps counteract the experience of worthlessness.

A young woman had come into analysis because of severe depression following a social rebuff by a community organization she had attempted to join. During treatment, it was very important to her to tell me about all her social successes, her children's achievements, her husband's professional honors, and her own many accomplishments. On one occasion, she proudly told me about how she had persuaded a friend to do something very difficult but beneficial and expected me to acknowledge her skill as well as the generosity of her effort. At the time, I was preoccupied with some other important issues in her analysis, and instead of interpreting her intense need for acknowledgment by me, I erroneously interpreted her denial of separation fears regarding her friend. Her response was icy, and when she returned for the next session, she reported having been extremely upset after the last session to the point that she "inadvertently" ran a red light on the way home. Selfobject dynamic: fragmentation following insufficient mirroring response.

Ideal Hungry Personality. Ideal hungry personalities can experience themselves as worthwhile only by finding selfobjects to whom they can look up and by whom they can feel accepted.

A man that I was treating suddenly became enraged with me when he found out that I was going abroad via a charter-airline flight. His need for an idealized selfobject was so intense that he needed to see me as superior to the type of people who take cheap charter flights. The sudden disappointment in the idealized selfobject temporarily fragmented his vulnerable self with the transformation of his healthy self-assertiveness into pathological rage.

Alter-ego Hungry Personality. Alter-ego hungry personalities need confirmation by being associated with another self whose appearance, opinions, and values they share.

An analysand, during a major part of his analysis, would become very upset when he detected that I had a different opinion from his own, no matter what the topic. Selfobject dynamic: confirmation of this fragile self required the selfobject to enact quite literally the image of the self's alter-ego.

Merger Hungry Personality. Merger hungry personalities need to control their selfobjects because they use them in lieu of self structure. Their need to control is often experienced by their selfobjects as a feeling of being oppressed, because the merger hungry person cannot bear the other's independence or separation from him or her.

Contact Shunning Personality. In contact shunning personalities, the intensity of their need for others is exceeded only by their sensitivity to the expected rejection. Therefore, isolating defenses come prominently into the foreground—not as symptomatic of lack of interest but, to the contrary, as symptoms of the widely excessive need. The two major defensive constellations here are schizoid or paranoid in appearance.

Schizoid defenses withdraw and hide the vulnerable self from the feared vicissitudes of social intercourse. Alternatively, paranoid defenses may surround the vulnerable self with such an aura of suspicion and hostility that potentially dangerous intruding selfobjects are held off at a safe distance.

ACTING OUT

The intense suffering associated with pathology of the self impellingly motivates toward amelioration by forcing the environment to yield the required comfort-giving experiences. Intensity of need combined with expectation of rebuff causes deep shame. Stridently expressed demands may alternate with total suppression of them. Demands, whether expressed in fantasy or in behavior, whether they are related to grandiosity or to being accepted by idealized figures, are not derived from the normal healthy self-assertive narcissism of childhood, but from the fragments of archaic selfobject needs or from the defenses against them.

Here is an example of a narcissistic behavior disorder:

A young artist felt compelled to "cruise" until he had made a homosexual pick-up whenever he experienced a faulty selfobject response from his coworkers. The quick sexual encounter would usually suffice to provide sufficient responsiveness to avoid fragmentation of the self even though no on-going relationship ever developed. Selfobject dynamic: Faulty selfobject response threatens self with fragmentation, which is avoided by "emergency" homosexual relation.

LIMITATIONS OF CLASSIFICATIONS

After having proceeded so blithely to present a nosological scheme to facilitate an orientation to the disorders of selfobject relations, it is necessary to point out and to warn that such systematic classifications are not to be taken as more than orienting and guiding frameworks. To be sure, the classic psychoanalytic typology of character into anal, oral, urethral, phallic, genital, and phallic–narcissistic characters suffers from similar shortcomings and should similarly not be used as a defining classification. There exist a number of difficulties that give rise to serious objections to almost any of the usual character nosologies. First of all, the simplified correlation of specific patterns of manifest behavior with universally present psychological conditions, which of necessity forms part of any such typology, will, in the long run, impede scientific progress.

Second, the impression is inevitably created, when presenting such a classification within a schema for ordering disorders, that the conditions so classified are, in fact, of a pathological nature. But that is plainly not true. Indeed, the constellations of structures that are designated as character-types vary in significance all the way from normal to severely pathological. The boundary between illness and health is vague and undetermined. The confusion originates from the fact that the sources of our conceptualizations are psychopathological phenomena.

Third, there is no stable correlation between etiological factors and the descriptive–phenomenological patterns. The behavior described as "mirror-hungry," for example, does not necessarily imply a deprivation of mirroring as the etiological agent. Only in the most general sense is it true that faulty selfobject relations during the formative stages of infancy and childhood will eventuate in adult behavior patterns that are characterized by faulty selfobject relations.

The complexity of human psychological experience no less than the complexity of human behavior are of such a degree that the precise representation in the exact formulations of scientific theories remains at present an elusive goal. This inescapable fact, however, does not significantly detract from the usefulness and epistemological soundness of the scientific theories that we create to order the chaos of observations in and around us. Similarly, the typologies to which we feel so attracted need not be shunned because of the limitations just discussed. But we should avoid going beyond their usefulness as direction-setting guides, and we should make sure that our misguided zeal for theorizing does not lead us into building fancy systems of thought unless the latter clearly articulate harmoniously with contemporary contiguous scientific fields.

.6.

NARCISSISTIC RAGE

RAGE IN INDIVIDUALS

In his essay "Of Anger," Michel de Montaigne talks about a passion that takes pleasure in itself and flatters itself. Manifesting his love for illustrating with stories from antiquity, Montaigne (1588) tells about Piso, a man of notable virtue in everything except his passionate anger, who became incensed at one of the men in his command. The soldier had returned alone from foraging and could give no account of where he had left a companion. Jumping to the conclusion that the soldier had murdered his companion, Piso promptly condemned him to death. At the last moment, with the soldier already at the gallows, the lost companion showed up. The army celebrated. The two comrades hugged and embraced, and the executioner took them to Piso, whom everyone confidently expected to experience the same great pleasure. The opposite happened. Piso's anger increased instead, and in his fury he condemned all three to death: the first soldier because there was a sentence against him; the second, who had been lost, because he was the cause of his companion's death, and the executioner for not having obeyed the command Piso had given him.

Let us now ask the origin of Piso's fury, which led to the death of three of his valued men. What can we say about this sudden unexpected outbreak of rage? Montaigne gives us a hint when he wonders that through shame and vexation Piso's fury made three guilty because he had found one innocent. The appearance of the lost companion had cleared the first soldier of guilt and thereby implied Piso to have been of rash and faulty judgment. To be seen publicly so defective was experienced as an unbearable narcissistic injury that could be healed only by eliminating the accusing presence. All three must be found guilty by any means or reason in order to restore Piso's narcissistic equilibrium. Only by effecting their death and disappearance could he remove the feeling of utter helplessness against being exposed to humiliating and self-destroying shame.

Passionate fury is one of the more frequent phenomena that arise out of the relations of humans with their surrounding world. Psychoanalysis has long recognized that aggression in its protean forms is as important a motivator of human action as is sexuality. The source and origin of the so-called aggressive drive had remained a matter of speculation. In a revision of his instinct theory, Freud (1920a) proposed two qualities of the mind: a self-destructive one, *thanatos* or death instinct, and an object-seeking one, *eros* or the life instinct. Aggression in all its forms, according to Freud, thus can be conceptualized as a manifestation of the death instinct. Most psychoanalysts, however, have not subscribed to Freud's philosophical reasoning. The concept of a death instinct has not found wide acceptance, and psychoanalysts generally prefer to talk about aggressive drives in analogy to the sexual drives. Clinical observations, moreover, frequently demonstrate a reactive character to aggression, because it is often seen in response to frustration.

Kohut (1972) extensively discussed the issues of human aggression and destructiveness. Kohut distinguishes two kinds of aggression—competitive aggressiveness, directed at objects that stand in the way of cherished goals, and narcissistic rage, directed at selfobjects who threaten or have damaged the self. For example, Montaigne's virtuous Piso was frustrated in his cherished goal of strengthening his army when he believed that his foraging team had failed by fighting with each other. His competitive aggressiveness was aroused at the surviving soldier of the foraging team, whom he condemned as an obstacle to the aim of a strong army, one competitively stronger than its potential opponents. But, much more seriously, Piso felt injured in his self-esteem when the returning companion made Piso appear to have been hasty and faulty in his judgment. This assault on his self aroused the narcissistic rage that could only be slaked by the disappearance of the offenders. When the selfobjects no longer fulfill their function of sustaining the self and, instead, make the self feel helpless, they must be eliminated. In Piso's case, the men who had made him look good now made him look foolish and thus were a threat to the cohesion of his self. They must be wiped off the face of the earth.

The two types of aggression—competitive aggressiveness and narcissistic rage—are structurally different and have very different psychological consequences. Competitive aggressiveness is a normal healthy reaction to obstacles that hinder the attainment of the person's aims in the world. Much of the energy with which we build and change the world is derived from competitive aggressiveness, which disappears spontaneously when the frustrating hurdle that evoked it has been overcome. No psychopathological residues remain in the wake of the vanished competitive aggressiveness. Even the experiences of intense competitiveness per se, for instance, in the context of the oedipus complex or in sibling rivalry, do not become the nucleus for psychoneuroses. It is always the nature of the selfobject response, whether it is being experienced as supportive or as threatening to the cohesion of the self, that determines a possible pathogenic effect. Thus, competitive aggressiveness derived from the oedipus complex is a nonpathological and often constructive force in human relations. If, however, the oedipal selfobjects respond to the oedipal child's sensual–competitive strivings with horror, or outrage, or derision, or rejection and humiliation, then the child's self is injured in its very core. "How can they do this to me?" the injured child asks noncomprehendingly. The frustrated sensuality will not disappear completely, but be repressed and return as a neurotic symptom. Similarly, the frustrated competitive aggressiveness and self-assertiveness will also reappear in neurotically distorted forms. The self's sensuality and assertiveness will manifest somehow, albeit in neurotically distorted or perverted form.

The real danger lies elsewhere. It arises when no self-assertion at all is possible, when the self feels absolutely helpless, vexed, and mortified, that is, paralyzed while agitated to the extreme and in deathly danger of losing its integrity. Such a self state is unbearable and must be altered. The offending selfobject or the totally ashamed self must be made to disappear, violently if necessary, even if the whole world will go up in flames.

A young man recalled his intense rivalrous competitiveness with a younger brother. He utterly resented that his brother was given special privileges, such as the tastiest morsels at the dinner table, and was allowed minor infractions of rules of conduct for which the older one was always reprimanded. He recalled enjoying a game that he had invented—obviously a compensatory structure—the essence of which consisted of his being the "policeman," complete with wearing a badge, who ordered his playmate brother to do all sorts of unpleasant chores. The younger one reluctantly complied, until finally he complained to his mother, who was incensed and angrily took away the "policeman's badge." In the analysis it became evident that what had remained as a festering sore in the adult's memory was not rivalrous rage with the brother nor the small favors the sibling had enjoyed, but the humiliating submission to having his badge confiscated. Even now, when he could rationalize that event as trivial, he still experienced it as so mortifying that he could hardly get himself to talk about it. He experienced the seizure of the badge as an assault on his self, because at that stage of his psychological development, the grandiose fantasy symbolized by the badge was an integral part of his self structure. Ever since this childhood incident he has been exquisitely sensitive to what he perceives as "injustice." Whether such "injustices" concern him directly or whether they occur in situations far removed from him, he is deeply disturbed by them. He then feels impelled to do something, often something foolishly inappropriate, such as telephoning strangers or writing outraged letters. These quixotic outbursts are fueled by narcissistic rage evoked when the so-called "injustices" make him feel utterly powerless.

In this particular young man, the capacity for creating compensatory structures determined that the psychopathology resulting from this trauma (in conjunction with many other analogous incidents) took the form of compensatory grandiose fantasies that never became integrated into healthy ambitions. Instead, his unintegrated grandiosity was expressed in a kind of arrogant behavior that led to his coming into analysis.

The origin of the narcissistic rage must be sought in the child-hood experience of utter helplessness *vis-à-vis* the humiliating self-object parent who robbed him unjustly of his badge. Such experiences of helplessness are unbearably painful, because they threaten the very continuity and existence of the self and they therefore evoke the strongest emergency defense of the self in the form of narcissistic rage. It has been my experience, when analyzing episodes of narcissistic rage that took the form of homicidal or suicidal fantasies, that they were almost invariably associated with intolerable experiences of helplessness in the face of an assault on the self.

Narcissistic rage does not vanish when the offending selfobject no longer exists. The painful memory lingers on, and so does the slowly boiling resentment. At some point, weeks, months, or even years after the insult, the smoldering animosity is likely to break out into open hostility, perhaps a hot fury, perhaps a coldly calculating destructiveness, and find its satisfaction in victimizing a substitute selfobject that has given offense. Severe narcissistic injuries sustained in childhood and experienced in a context of unendurable helplessness may thus give the personality forever the pathological cast of a chronic paranoid character formation.

A conceptual comprehension of the development of normal assertiveness and competitiveness of the self as well as the selfobject experiences that lead to narcissistic rage is a prerequisite to rational psychoanalytic treatment. Even intense rivalries and competitive aggressiveness directed at frustrating objects are not pathological per se, whether they manifest extra-analytically or in the transference. There is little need for interpretation unless such behaviors carry an admixture of selfobject-directed narcissistic rage. For example, the burdens engendered by the psychoanalytic situation, with its constraints of time and place that sometimes seriously interfere with other important goals of the analysand, may cause some irritation and annoyance. These frustrations, however, usually pass easily. Other aspects of the psychoanalytic situation, especially when certain technical precepts are applied rigidly—for example, an exaggerated technical neutrality or excessively prolonged silences—are often experienced as deprivations of legitimate and necessary selfobject responses. The self's structure weakens in the absence of the needed responsiveness. Feeling assaulted, the self may turn on the selfobject in narcissistic rage, particularly if the deprivation experienced during treatment is linked to the pathogenic past by appearing to be a repetition of it in the present. Such disruptions (cf. Chapter 9) may become an occasion for the restoration of the self through explanations and interpretation, or they may lead to a precipitous termination of treatment if their severity destroys the selfobject tie with the therapist.

Narcissistic rage is seen in narcissistic personality disorders, but most frequently in borderline patients. In the latter, the tenuousness of their selfobject ties, including their tie to the therapist, always makes these episodes of narcissistic rage a threat to the treatment process. But even when treatment continues, it remains a difficult task to achieve an amelioration of the rage. Interpretation usually has little effect, because it is not experienced as supportive to the self. Indeed, interpretations are often experienced as criticisms that aggravate the self's vulnerability. What the self needs is to be understood. However, that does not mean the self needs approval of its rage. It may take a very long period of time during which empathic understanding alone rules before a gradual fading away of the rage takes place.

THE RAGE OF GROUPS

I want to digress briefly from my primary focus on the clinical aspects of self psychology, that is, the psychological treatment of individuals. Narcissistic rage is also a group phenomenon of such importance that any contribution self psychology might make to our understanding justifies this detour.

The group phenomena that I have in mind are not those terrible impacts that the violent actions of a narcissistically enraged person can have on small or large groups of people. The terror created when an individual throws a bomb into a crowd deserves serious discussion at some other time. Neither am I proposing to review the contributions that self psychology has made to the study of the relationship between the narcissistic rage of charismatic or messianic leaders and group psychology (cf. Kohut, 1976; Wolf, 1976b). To be sure, there is a place for the self-psychological study of organized groups as well as of crowd behavior under extreme conditions. In the following, however, I am more interested in the concept of a "group self" (Kohut, 1976, p. 419f) and its relation to narcissistic rage.

As a first step in this discussion, we have to perform the difficult maneuver of thinking about an organized group as if it were an individual. Introspection and empathy can come to our aid in making us aware of the close relationship between aspects of our personal identity and that of the group to which we belong. For example, to the extent that we as individuals are identified with our country, we feel proud when the United States achieves some remarkable success, perhaps the fulfilment of some great ambition in the face of seemingly insuperable obstacles—sending men to the moon and back comes to mind—or the country's attempt to live up to its lofty ideals of freedom for all. Clearly, at such moments, we know with great certainty that the United States and its people as a group has, consciously or perhaps unconsciously, a set of commonly shared ambitions and ideals which are independent of the ambitions and ideals of its individual citizens, though the latter may and sometimes do share in them. Is it, then, too mystical to conjecture that these demonstrable ambitions and ideals of the group are constitutive of a group self? Let us then assume that a cohesive group has a group self in analogy to cohesively organized individuals. The phenomenon that is known by the term *esprit de corps* (the regard entertained by the members of a body for the honor and interests of the body as a whole, and of each other as belonging to it, as the *Oxford English Dictionary* defines it) recognizes the special relationship between a group self and the selfs of its constituents. Self psychology therefore has something useful to say about some of the various psychological states of such group selfs. And, perhaps, from the observed behavior of some groups we might be able to make inferences about their group selfs, which may, on the one hand, confirm some of our conjectures, and, on the other hand, be of some practical usefulness.

As an illustrative example let us look at the Arab–Israeli conflict. A truly neutral outside observer might be excused for thinking that these two great and intelligent peoples ought to be able to negotiate a rational way of living together in peace and freedom, each according to their own aims and values. But like individuals, groups have a history that has shaped their hopes and their fears and distorted their ambitions and ideals. One need not be a historian or specialist on the Middle East to have some sense of the glorious past of the Arab people who marched from victory to victory, conquering most of the then known world while the West was still in the Dark Ages. The Arabs brought with them not only pacification and prosperity, but also the cultural traditions of the ages, including the wisdom of the ancients of East and West. This splendid past was then brought into a precipitous decline by—in all honesty we must admit—hordes of barbarians pouring out of the northwest corner of Europe. Adding insult to injury, these barbarians, during subsequent centuries, by basing themselves on the philosophy and science of the Greeks that had been transmitted to them by the Arabs, built our powerful modern technological civilization, while the proud Arabs gradually found themselves reduced to the relative poverty and powerlessness of vassals. Only in this century, fueled by the power of oil and the ideals of democracy, has an Arab nationalism begun to restore the cohesion of its formerly grand self. And then, as if out of nowhere, the West suddenly establishes in their midst, like a colonial enclave, the state of Israel. It should not be surprising that the Arab self feels threatened in its very existence and reacts with narcissistic rage to the perception of vulnerability and helplessness.

On the other side, the Jews, have a history as a people that is no less magnificent than that of the Arabs. Although the martial accomplishments of the Jewish group self were more limited and in the distant past, their group self compensated for lost political ambitions by a grandiose fantasy of being special—the chosen people—and, in compensation for their shrunken ambitions, by letting their ideals hypertrophy into a scholarly morality with a messianic fervor. But the political powerlessness, underlined by pogroms and holocaust, remained a constant threat to the cohesion and the survival of the Jewish self. Then, suddenly, as a result of unique circumstances arising from World War II, the age-old ambition to return to Jerusalem and restore a strong and cohesive group self was achieved. For the first time in two thousand years, Jews can be proud to be part of the Jewish nation again, to be part of Israel. They cannot relinquish this restored healthy and cohesive group self without fragmenting. By surrendering the newly won status of being an ordinary people in its land like any other, they would inevitably return to the pathologically narcissistic fantasy of being the chosen ones. Can they possibly give up their country and return to feeling weak and despised because they lack a cohesive and strong group self? Such are the questions that deeply agitate the Jewish people, that threaten the very existence of the Jewish group self, and evoke the increasingly shrill and rageful responses.

Self psychology has no easy answers to the issues posed by the narcissistic vulnerabilities and rages of group selfs. It seems inescapable, however, that threats and other weakening maneuvers cause a self's sense of helplessness to increase and with it the intensity of the evoked narcissistic rage. One is left with the seemingly paradoxical suggestion that real peace—not the peace of surrender but the peace of mutual empathic understanding—comes from strengthening, not weakening, the enemy's self.

For a discussion, in the light of selfobject theory, of the relations between leaders and groups, see Chapter 3, pages 48-49.

. II .

TREATMENT

.7.

THE SETTING

SITUATION, AMBIENCE, AND PROCESS

The psychoanalytic endeavor takes place in a psychoanalytic setting. The psychoanalytic *situation*, the psychoanalytic *ambience*, and the psychoanalytic *process* designate three different aspects of the clinical psychoanalytic setting. All three are so closely intermeshed that change in one is usually accompanied by changes in the other two as well. But a differentiation of the psychoanalytic situation from the psychoanalytic ambience and from the psychoanalytic process will clarify our thinking about each one of these aspects of clinical psychoanalysis and how they affect one another.

By psychoanalytic situation I mean the *participants*, that is, analyst and analysand, the arrangements of time, place, fees, and other obligations and, in general, anything observable and reportable by an outside party. At times it may also be interesting and germane to ask how the psychoanalytic situation appears to nonparticipants, for example, to spouses, friends, relatives, third-party providers, and the genreal public. The situation, then, is viewed from an objective-interpersonal perspective.

By psychoanalytic ambience I mean to designate how the psychoanalytic situation is *experienced* by the participants. The ambience is viewed from a subjective-intrapsychic perspective. Therefore, the ambience is likely to be experienced differently by the analysand than by the analyst.

Finally, the psychoanalytic process designates the presumably lawful *psychological changes* initiated and maintained by the participants in the psychoanalytic endeavor by virtue of their participation. Conceptually, one may distinguish two different intrapsychic psychoanalytic processes: one in the analysand and one in the analyst. In practice, we are mostly concerned with the process that has been initiated in the analysand and that eventually—we hope—will lead to an analysis of his or her self by that self. We are interested in the process that has been activated in the analyst only to the extent that it might hinder or facilitate the analytic process in the analysand by affecting the analyst's conduct in the analytic setting, that is, the countertransference reactions.

The aim of the clinical psychoanalytic endeavor is to initiate and maintain a psychoanalytic process. Strange as it may seem, however, the psychoanalytic endeavor does not aim to end the process that it seeks to initiate; in fact, a successful conclusion of the mutual endeavor of analyst and analysand is indicated by the continuance of the process, albeit within each individual, without further facilitation from the other. Let it be noted at this point that this self-analytic process would ideally continue for both analyst and analysand ad infinitum, even after any formal relationship between them has ceased.

Analyst and analysand can anticipate that they will be working with each other for a number of years. The workplace, therefore, should be quiet, comfortable, and neither luxurious nor austere. Analytic neutrality does not require the clean sterility of the laboratory; analysts inevitably reveal aspects of their style, taste, and other personal predilections. Patients know that their analysts are human beings with idiosyncratic interests. Trying to pretend otherwise is bound to fail sooner or later. But, worse, attempting to be someone other than oneself contradicts the whole spirit of the analytic endeavor, which, I believe, is to acknowledge and strengthen the self and its self expression.

The analyst should furnish his or her consulting room in harmony with his or her aesthetic preferences and intellectual interests. Ambiguous invisibility is not a necessary precondition for the emergence of intense transferences, nor does the presence of the analyst as a real person inhibit the transference relation. Indeed, the analyst is a real person who likes and dislikes and who unavoidably manifests his or her personality in his or her office and personal decor, thus evoking certain transference reactions that can be recognized and interpreted. There is no need for the analyst to pretend being anonymous and ambiguous like a Rorschach ink blot. The analyst cannot hide, yet should not intrude beyond visibly and audibly stating his or her presence. By implication the analyst thus announces his or her availability as a potential carrier for the selfobject function without forcing himself or herself upon the analysand. A reasonable regard for protecting his or her own privacy will underline the analyst's determination to similarly protect the privacy of his or her ment of my position is in order. I have chosen to practice psycho-analysis because this method of psychological treatment appears to be the most suitable method for certain patients that come to me as a physician specializing in psychiatry. In general, I find myself in harmony with the traditional ethics of medical practice. I recognize that patients consult psychoanalysts because they are experiencing psychological pain and have the hope that psychoanalysis will ameliorate their suffering. In accepting such patients as analysands, I express my belief that there exists a reasonable expectation of their finding some alleviation of their discomfort through psychoanalysis, and I agree to make this presumed goal of the patient the overriding aim of the joint analytic endeavor. I realize that some patients' unhappiness is reflected in their behavior, and that often these patients seek to alter their behavior with the help of psychoanalytic therapy. However, psychological methods of treatment are limited by their very nature to strengthening the patient's self through the experiences and understanding gained as part of the psychoanalytic treatment process. The psychoanalyst, therefore, cannot presume to alter another person's behavior except by helping him or her to be stronger and understand himself or herself better. Nevertheless, the patient's goals remain the final justification for the treatment effort. Other goals, such as the facilitation of the patient's comprehension of his or her mental life and behavior—although of great importance to the psychoanalyst—are merely instrumental and subordinated to the overall well-being of the patient. A common belief among many psychoanalysts holds that an analyst's therapeutic ambition is detrimental to the success of the psychoanalytic venture. I regard this belief as false; it contradicts the very function of a psychological physician in our culture. Such apparent contradictions derive from differences in the definition of the goal of a clinical psychoanalysis. Traditionally, this goal has been defined mainly in terms of the patient's knowledge of himself rather than in terms of his experience of himself. The idea has been that the quest for psychological truth should be the foremost guide, and that the therapeutic results, when possible, will follow almost automatically.

For a number of reasons, a definition of the task of clinical psychoanalysis that refers only to the truth of the patient's knowledge of himself, and not also to his affective state and experience of himself, is unacceptable to me. There is very little evidence that a facilitation of the patient's knowledge of his mental life and behavior will in itself increase his sense of well-being. On the contrary, I have observed—and I think most psychoanalysts can corroborate this observation—some postanalytic patients who were well "analyzed" but not cured: They had achieved wide and deep knowledge about the dynamics of their conscious and unconscious mental functioning but had not benefited to any significant extent from a lasting amelioration of their psychological pain nor from any meaningful improvement in their unhappy relations with others. It is too easy to dismiss these unfortunate cases by saying they were not really analyzed, when indeed they did gain a markedly better comprehension of their mental life. Perhaps, with many of these patients, nothing more ambitious can be achieved, and certainly, no psychoanalyst should promise more. But such analyses fall short of the goals with which the patient came into treatment, and we should not hesitate to call them failures.

On the other hand, we can also observe patients who seem to garner very little reportable self-knowledge in their analyses and who after termination can hardly remember what happened. Many of these patients clearly feel better, function better, are more creative and happier in their relationships. These may be patients who have achieved—to speak conceptually—an uninterrupted tension arc from the pole of ambitions to the pole of ideals and are thus enabled, perhaps for the first time, to enact their nuclear program in a self-satisfying productive and creative fashion. Are we to say that they had a good therapeutic result but were not really analyzed? I prefer a definition of the goals of clinical psychoanalysis that does not slight the patient's goal of an improved sense of well-being and an improved overall functioning. By making the patient's experience of himself, his functioning, and his relations with others the touchstone by which the analytic achievement will be measured, I make no implied promise that we will necessarily reach that goal. Indeed, most of the time we must be satisfied with small increments of improvement, but these will be improvements that can be appreciated by the patient, and not just by the analyst. Such improvements may be small on some scale, but have the most significant and beneficial impact on the patient's life.

From the beginning, therefore, the emphasis is on the subjective experience of the analysand rather than on so-called objective assessments by criteria emanating from outside the analysand's self-experience. There are pitfalls in such a commitment to the analysand's self-centered view of himself. The dangers of solipsistic illusions entered into by the patient and supported by the analyst are obvious. In this book, most of the substance of the numerous technical questions about conducting a psychoanalysis make strengthening the analysand's self its primary goal without at the same time falling into the trap of mutually shared illusions.

However, at this point I wish to touch on the rarely discussed relationship of society to this rather precious twosome, the analyst and the analysand, in their very private analytic cocoon. It is a measure of the strength and maturity of a society when it can tolerate and even support in its midst an encapsulated precinct of commitment to just one individual. I have previously noted (Wolf, 1980a) that

> I can approach the ethics of medical practice only from the point of view of my own commitment to the primacy of the individual who comes to the physician for help. I am fortunate that the society in which I live and work allows me and my patients this privileged corner where my patient's innermost and private goals, whether conscious or unconscious, can, by and large, be freely explored. And I am totally convinced that the well-being of that society depends, in large measure, on its willingness to encourage enclaves, such as my consulting room, where it is not necessarily the values of the group but those of the individual that prevail. (pp. 43–44)

All these considerations, however, still miss the point for many patients, who are not particularly interested in the analyst's values and ethics nor in his or her professional commitments. Such patients are unhappy because they feel unloved and unlovable—in fact, they usually were unloved as children and did become unlovable as a result—and they demand, more or less covertly, that the therapist prove that he or she really cares. The psychoanalyst who insists that the best and only service he or she can perform for the patient is to analyze is likely to be misunderstood and to lose those patients who experience such an explicit analytic posture as not caring. Many times such treatments will drag on for months or even years before the participants face up to the sad fact that they are operating at cross-purposes.

But will the treatment fare any better if the therapist decides to demonstrate to the patient in word and deed that he or she really is concerned? Unfortunately, the chances for successful treatment are little better with the expressly caring therapist. Love is not enough, because there is never enough love. The present cannot undo the past. What hope is there for such stalemated treatments? Should the analyst implicitly hold out the hope that the patient's goal of feeling better about himself and his world is attainable through finding a substitute, even if more or less illusory, for the missing parental love? Or should the patient be told about the impossibility of his quest and be encouraged to reduce his expectations to a realistically more achievable level?

Apparently the answers to these questions depend on the analyst's value system, on whether he or she believes the most important value is to care for what happens to another human being, or whether the analyst deems the truth, as best as he or she can determine it, as the highest value. I believe much of the animosity between various analytic groups—for example, the accusation that one is soft and perhaps doing good psychotherapy but poor analysis, or, on the other hand that one is cold and unempathically indifferent to human suffering—is derived more from conflicting value systems than from different theories. Viewed from the point of view of a scientific depth psychology, that is, psychoanalysis, the conflict is a spurious one. I hope to be able to demonstrate that the choice is not between empathy or truth, but rather that the psychoanalyst can and should be committed to both. The analyst can appreciate why the patient who was or felt deprived of the needed parental care during childhood is now demanding the analyst's utmost concern. In trying to understand the patient's past and present, the analyst accepts the patient as he or she is without making any demands for change. Indeed, the analyst is not concerned with either loving the patient now or whether the patient's past experience actually happened that way or not. The analyst simply tries to accept, understand, and explain as best he or she can, and always not nearly as well as the patient expects. If the patient, in spite of painful disappointments, can also come to accept the analyst with his or her shortcomings, then a psychoanalytic process will establish itself and will likely be blessed also with the patient's experience of an improved sense of well-being.

.8.

PRINCIPLES

UNDOING THE EFFECTS OF INJURY TO THE SELF

Treating, healing, restoring, and curing are all terms that have found favor at some time or other for the process of undoing the effects that past psychological traumas can have in the present. No one, of course, can change the past. No substitute experience can undo now what happened in the past, nor can it remove the emotional scars left behind. Strengthening the self in the therapeutic situation by empathic resonance with the therapist, however, allows the self to reexperience the same old trauma now in a changed context. That changed context is provided by a self strengthened through experiencing the therapist as a selfobject. Changing the experiential context also changes the meaning of an experience and thus may make it possible to gradually loosen and discard the defensive armor acquired earlier in life to protect a modicum of self structure and functioning. The therapeutic regression of the self, which is engendered by the treatment situation, makes the self's structure more fluid and thus makes the self again more adaptable to changing experiences. Distorted aspects of the self's experience of itself and of others come into renewed contact with a different reality, which it may experience as benign, learn to understand, and to which it may then gradually readapt itself.

The therapeutic process just outlined is predicated, among other factors, on the self being sufficiently strong to withstand the process. The self must be strong enough to withstand, especially, the therapeutic regression and the painful disruptions of the transference, without further uncontrolled and undue regression or total and perhaps irreversible fragmentation of the self. Patients who never achieved a cohesive self, therefore, are not suitable for psychoanalytic treatment. This eliminates most of the functional psychoses—in particular, schizophrenia and the severe dysthymic disorders—from psychoanalysis as a treatment method. Though the lack of a cohesive

self is covered over by defenses in the borderline states, these patients are also disposed to regress severely with loss of structure. As a
rule, they are not analyzable, though this is difficult to predict; the
final diagnosis should not be based on any kind of theoretical definition or brief clinical assessment, but only on a sufficient trial and
failure of psychoanalytic treatment.

Weak Self at Center of Pathology

Certain principles should be restated. A weakened self stands at
the center of all selfobject relations disorders. Therefore, the treatment process should aim at strengthening the self. Strengthening
the self takes precedence over all other possible aims, for example,
making the unconscious conscious, remembering, reconstructing, resolving conflict, and the like. These latter aims are important also,
but they usually become possible to the strengthened self without the
need for specific measures.

A weak self is the result of faulty selfobject experiences. The
vulnerability of a weak self disposes it to certain self-defeating
defenses that lead to difficulties with potential sources of enhancing
selfobject experiences. As a consequence of these difficult and frustrating experiences with the available selfobjects, the vulnerable
self's needs are not adequately met and lead to further weakening of
the self. A vignette will illustrate:

A forty-five-year-old professional man came into treatment because of
chronic depression. As the only child of elderly parents, he was doted on by
an overprotective mother who effectively prevented him from participating
in the rough-and-tumble of playing with his peers. Instead, he was given
much encouragement and profuse approbation for intellectual activities of
all kinds in which he, indeed, excelled. From the point of view of the
parents, this was not only reasonable—after all, why should he risk getting
hurt playing with those roughnecks when he could spend that time enjoying
good reading and good music?—but also suited the aged parents' low
tolerance for the confusing noisiness of children and adolescents. The
youngster thus grew up in compliance with his parents' needs, while his
own needs for gratifying selfobject experiences evoked by pleasure in the
effectiveness of his body and by self-enhancing selfobject experiences with
his peer group were greatly curtailed. No one admired him, only certain

parts of him were acceptable to others, and consequently his self lacked cohesion and was prone to fragmentation. A resulting sense of both physical and social inadequacy were symptomatic of this vulnerability. To keep from regressing further, he engaged in certain sexualized rituals and obsessive preoccupations that distracted him from the ever-present sense of inadequacy. He yearned for the selfobject experiences, particularly with his peer group, that were so needed for the strengthening of his self. But the very defenses of intellectualization and a certain haughtiness that protected his self-esteem simultaneously interfered with peer relations and thus led to further deprivation. He became a loner—talented, moody, living in fantasy, deprived of the self-sustaining selfobject experiences of an active social life.

At the extreme, a weakened self is in danger of regressing to total fragmentation, that is, to dissolution and death. Persons with weakened selfs are, more or less, aware of their weakness and sense some of the dangers to which they are exposed as a consequence. Symptoms such as anxiety or excessive irritability warn of the impending threat to the self. People with weak selfs suffer unpleasant symptoms in great discomfort or act out unacceptable behaviors. They come into treatment with the hope of being helped.

A weakened self may be weak for one or more of three reasons: (1) because faulty selfobject experiences during crucial developmental periods interfered with the normally unfolding developmental processes and development became arrested in one or more particular sectors of the developing self; (2) because of injury sustained as a result of faulty selfobject relations during the developmental phases, mostly in childhood, but also during certain developmental crises such as adolescence, midlife, and aging; and (3) because the fragility of a vulnerable self forces it into defensive postures that interfere with current selfobject relationships and thus effectively hinder the establishment of self-sustaining and self-healing selfobject experiences in the here-and-now.

Strengthening the Weak Self

Rational treatment, therefore, should address itself to strengthening the weak self, if possible. This strengthening of the self comes about via the psychoanalytic process, which in a step-wise fashion replaces the archaic (and thus pathological) needs for selfobject responses with age-appropriate needs for selfobject responses—that is, replaces the archaic needs with a selfobject response that we might label reciprocal empathic resonance. Without at this time going into the technical details for activating the psychoanalytic process, let me outline the steps as follows.

By providing a proper ambience of noninterference, the therapist is enabled to interpret resistances to treatment—that is, fears—allowing and facilitating the emergence of the archaic selfobject needs in the treatment situation (cf. Shane, 1985). The emerging selfobject needs will spontaneously focus on the therapist; that is, a selfobject transference develops. This transference will be disrupted, often very painfully, when inevitably the therapist somehow fails to respond in precisely the manner required by the patient. The therapist then explains and interprets this disruption in all its dimensions, but particularly with reference to analogous early and presumably etiological situations with significant persons of the past. These explanations and interpretations restore the previous harmonious selfobject transference, but the mutual understanding achieved and experienced thereby serves to replace the previously frustrated archaic selfobject need with a reciprocal empathic resonance with the therapist, which strengthens the self. The selfobject experience with the therapist strengthens the self, and it becomes better able to integrate into a social selfobject matrix, that is, to successfully find responsive selfobject experiences in the social surround unhampered by defenses.

NEUTRALITY AND ABSTINENCE

Abstinence is one of the rules of psychoanalytic technique, though, as Rycroft (1968, p. 1) tells us, it is not clear what the patient should be made to abstain from. Freud stressed that the analyst not gratify the patient's demands for love, but he did not hesitate to feed the Wolf Man when needed, and the reports from Freud's analysands testify to his being anything but formal, cold, and stiffly detached.

A rational approach would prescribe that the patient abstain from whatever interferes with the therapeutic process. This means that both patient and therapist should abstain from turning the professional relationship into an ordinary social relationship.

Clearly, the pleasures of social intimacy of all degrees will distract from the analytic work and tempt both patient and therapist to avoid the pain of re-experiencing traumatic memories. Social intimacy, therefore, must be avoided. However, that does not mean a rigid adherence to rules of analytic etiquette, but a flexible freedom to respond to each other as friendly and interested human beings. Such freedom would include expressing one's condolences at afflictions or bereavement, and expressing one's congratulations on appropriately happy occasions. Abstaining from the ordinary courtesies of friendly human discourse creates an impression of artificiality and lack of honesty that may well be destructive to the conduct of the therapeutic enterprise. It not only misleads the patient into thinking the therapist coldly detached and uninterested in the patient's affective experiences, but also sees to it that the patient experiences the therapist as unresponsive and uncaring. Such abstinence destroys the therapeutic ambience.

Traditionally, abstaining from any kind of gratification—as part of the technical neutrality of the analyst in the analytic situation—has been made into a technical prescription for doing analysis. According to Leider (1983, p. 665) neutrality is both an attitude and a technical stance most frequently recommended for the analyst, and many consider it essential to the definition of analytic treatment. These clinicians recommend that the analyst's proper function is to understand and to convey that understanding to the patient. In this view, neutrality requires adherence to the rule of abstinence, and a perspective equidistant from the demands of the id, ego, and superego. Such a neutrality insists on the exclusion of values other than the search for knowledge, of attitudes other than professional commitment, and of interventions other than interpretations.

From a self-psychological point of view, the proper attitude is more complex. The self psychologist emphasizes the importance of the re-experience in the transference of the archaic selfobject needs. Thus, the proper criteria for neutrality—or for abstinence or ambience—are determined by the optimal facilitation of this therapeutically useful re-experience. The patient will not give up his resistances because the analyst tells him to or because the analyst interprets them to him. The patient gives up his resistances slowly and gradually and cautiously when he has learned to trust the analyst a little bit. Some patients are never able to develop this degree of trusting and therefore they are the most difficult to treat. Those that learn to trust do so because they have gained the conviction that the therapist's neutrality is a friendly one, that is, that the therapist is affectively on the side of the patient's self without, however, necessarily joining the patient in all his judgments. It is one of the paradoxes of analytic therapy that once the patient has learned to trust the therapist and himself enough to really follow the basic rule of speaking without much censoring himself (it usually takes years of analytic work to reach this freedom from defensiveness), the analytic process has reached the point where the therapist is needed less and the analysis of the self by the self can proceed unaided much of the time.

INTERVENTIONS

Understanding is a good term for the process that is often referred to by a variety of synonyms, for example, being in tune with, attunement, or empathy. As stated earlier, Freud used the term *Einfuehlung*, which means to feel oneself into the subjective experience of another. The process of understanding is more than trying to figure out what another person is experiencing, because it is more than just a conscious, logical, cognitive process. To understand means to sense oneself into another's experience, that is, it includes preconscious and unconscious perceptions, particularly of affects. The term *affect attunement* used by infant researchers (Stern, 1985, pp. 138–161) seems to designate a process that is similar to what analysts call empathy. Analysts do not seem able to agree on a precise definition of empathy or to say much about the nature of what is involved; therefore, I will avoid trying to define with scientific precision a concept that is known well enough operationally. Clinically, I think, we all know what we mean when we say that somebody is empathic or in tune. This may be why Freud[1] could state that without empathy there cannot be any real understanding of another, yet never bothered to define empathy within his metapsychology. I will adhere to Kohut's usage, which distinguishes an initial affective *understanding* from a supplementary and more cognitively logical *explanation*. An empathic grasp, then, encompasses both understanding and explaining.

To explain is to provide a logical and verbal expression that will make intelligible a meaning for the observed phenomena.

1. "A path leads from identification by way of imitation to empathy, that is, to the comprehension of the mechanism by means of which we are enabled to take up any attitude at all towards another mental life" (Freud, 1921, *Standard Edition* 18:110, note 2).

To interpret is to bring out the meaning, that is, to explain within the frame of a specific theory. For example, an interpretation may be an explanation in terms of a psychoanalytic theory.

To enact is to express in an interpersonal context the meaning of an unconscious or preconscious communication by way of a more or less dramatized interaction.

Not Content, but the Experience

It is not the content of the information conveyed to the patient, not the substance of the interpretations and interventions made, not the correctness of the therapist's conjectures, nor even the therapist's compliance with demands to "mirror" the patient or to be his or her ideal that is pivotal: It is decisive for the progress of the therapeutic endeavor that the patient experience an ambience in which he or she feels respected, accepted, and at least a little understood.

This does not mean that the messages or information contained in communications and interpretations are unimportant. On the contrary, the correctness of interpretation is second only to the proper ambience in moving the analytic process forward. The informational content of an interpretation, however, will not be heard in depth unless given in an ambience that allows the patient to listen. More important than the ability to conceptualize his or her insights is the therapist's ability to sense the patient's need for the particular kind of ambience in which this therapy can proceed. The person who is the therapist thus becomes as crucial a variable as the person who is the patient.

Evocation of Mutative Experience

Clinical experience demonstrates that the knowledge gained by a patient about himself or herself has a certain usefulness to the patient, but does not effect any deep-going changes. Such new knowledge may have some influence on the patient's consciously controlled thinking and behavior, but it has no effect on unconscious experience. Reading self-improvement literature accomplishes few psychological changes even when the material convinces the reader. Similarly, the information conveyed by a therapist to a patient, let us say in an interpretation, has little significant impact. In order for an interpretation to be effective in causing change—to be mutative—it has to evoke an experience in the patient. What aspects of a therapeutic experience make it mutative?

First, the experience must involve the transference, that is, it must be an experience that involves intense feelings about the therapist, and these feelings must be related to the feelings associated with some traumatic events involving significant persons of the patient's early life. Second, to make the re-experience of the archaic affects in the here-and-now therapeutically effective and mutative, they must occur in a context where the patient understands and fully accepts both the actions and the affects of the therapist as well as his or her own. In other words—and this is the decisive difference when compared with the archaic situation—in the therapeutic situation, no blame is attached to either patient or therapist for the painful interactions that are taking place. They are accepted because they can be understood as occurring naturally, perhaps even inevitably. It is in this sense that knowledge of self and other—perhaps provided by an explanation or interpretation—can facilitate the experiential acceptance of painful interactions. The skillful interpreter establishes a link between the experience-near events in the here-and-now, the more distant events of the experienced archaic past, and the experience-distant explanations derived from general knowledge, history, and psychological theory. But sealing a mutative experience into a context by interpretation must be preceded by the evocation of the experience.

.9.

THE THERAPEUTIC PROCESS

In this section, I will elaborate the process by which an analysand (or a patient or a client) may achieve an improved state of mental health from the point of view of self psychology. In Kohut's view (1984, p. 7), the psychological health of the core of the personality is always best defined in terms of structural completeness, that is, in terms of an energic continuum in the center of the personality having been established such that the unfolding of a productive life has become a realizable possibility. Clearly, health is not merely a static condition. Implied in Kohut's definition is a view of the person embedded in a net of ever-changing relationships, the selfobject experience of which has evoked and maintained a structurally complete, vigorous, balanced and ever-changing self. In short, a healthy self is strong and creatively acting in community with others.

AIMS

Strengthening the Self

The ultimate aim of the therapeutic process should be to strengthen the self so that the person is willing and able to actively plunge into the rough-and-tumble of everyday life, not without fear, but nevertheless undeterred. The intermediate aim is to initiate an analytic process, and a long-term aim is to keep the analytic process active—optimally even beyond the termination of the formal therapeutic relationship—with the expected concomitant benefit of a strengthened self. Other aims are secondary to the primary aim of strengthening the self. Depending on one's theoretical conceptualization of health and pathology, the definition of the aims of treatment varies. Among the goals proposed at various times in the history of psychoanalytic practice have been: making the unconscious conscious, resolving unconscious conflicts, recovering a complete and truthful personal history, removing disturbing symptoms, controlling undesirable behavior, integrating into a social matrix, freeing potential creativity, reaching higher levels of maturity in development, improving the quality and depth of interpersonal relationships, improving the capacity to love and to work, and many more. All these goals are still laudable, but from the point of view of self psychology, what is not entailed in the aim of strengthening the self must be regarded as secondary to it.

The Goal of Treatment

The goal of treatment in self psychology has been described in structural terms as increasing the cohesion and wholeness of the self through transmuting internalization. As growing knowledge of the self disorders has enhanced our understanding, we have placed greater emphasis on the crucial vicissitudes of the selfobject experience. Empathic resonance with a responsive selfobject matrix is now seen as the guarantor of psychological structure and well-being. But whether the goal of treatment is defined in terms of self-structure (*i.e.*, restoration of the structural deficit or the establishment of an uninterrupted tension are from basic ambitions, via basic talents and skills, toward basic ideals)[1] or in terms of the selfobject milieu (*i.e.*, the ability to allow free and nonanxious closeness to a needed selfobject milieu), the result sought is a strengthening of the self's structure concomitant with a greater latitude in tolerating less than optimal selfobject experiences without a significant loss of self cohesion. No longer is it legitimate to demand that patients change. Instead, we can hold out the hope that the transmuting experiences of self-psychologically oriented treatment will enhance the strength of their self, and that in consequence of the incremental accretion of structure they will be able to integrate previously unintegrated affects.[2]

A patient's self is strengthened by re-experiencing the archaic trauma, with its associated affects, in the here-and-now of a therapeutic situation that allows an integrating and self-enhancing re-structuring of the self. This is not a corrective emotional re-experience as Alexander (1958, pp. 326-331) described it, because

1. cf. Kohut, 1984, p. 4.
2. Stolorow, Brandchaft, and Atwood, 1987, pp. 74-86.

the therapist is just as imperfect in his or her responsiveness as the parent was in childhood. Therefore, the therapist does not attempt to play a role that makes him or her different from the parent of childhood, as Alexander suggested. Indeed, the therapist's imperfection, that, is, his or her faulty responsiveness is as inevitable as the patient's experience of a painful disappointment and subsequent disruption in the empathic tie to the therapist. This is how there comes about a repetition of the traumatic experience of childhood in the here-and-now of the analytic situation. But the restoration of the disrupted tie through empathic understanding and explanation confers enough extra strength to the self to enable it to integrate the contents and affects of the traumatic disruption into the structure of the self. The self thus emerges from the disruption–restoration incrementally strengthened by having integrated into the organization of its self-experience the contents and affects of the disruption–restoration experience.

What distinguishes these wholesome therapeutic experiences from the disintegrating (disposing toward fragmentation) pathogenic experiences of the past? A number of factors can be mentioned here. There is the greater age and resilience of the more mature self. There is also, in analysis, the memory of many such previous disruption–restoration incidents that were repaired with gradually increasing trust in the therapist. But more importantly, there is the therapist's acceptance of the patient's reactions, including the demands and symptoms secondary to the fragmentation of the patient's self. The therapist knows that these behaviors are inevitable, given the patient's history and therefore subsequent weaknesses of the self that were brought into the therapeutic situation. The therapist does not ask the patient to change, as a parent might, but explains to the patient what is going on, with the hope that gradually the patient will continue to become stronger and therefore less reactive, that is, less disrupted.

In other words, the reason that the patient grows stronger in the therapeutic situation is that the therapist's rational equanimity signals an affective ambience of acceptance to the patient. In this ambience the patient's affects are able to calm down rather than being further exacerbated as they would be if the therapist responded with affectively colored nonacceptance of what the patient was experiencing. To put this into more technical language, the proper therapeutic ambience, by virtue of providing a selfobject matrix in which

the patient's self can become embedded, is experienced as an empathic resonance that is sufficiently strengthening to the cohesiveness of the self. The self's capacity for integrating the evoked unpleasant affects are enhanced without trauma to the self's structure
and cohesion and with an incremental accretion of structure.

Wish to Change?

It is often thought that successful treatment requires that the
patient have a strong wish to change. In the face of the difficulties
and obstacles attending psychoanalytic treatment, it seems only reasonable to expect that strong motivation is needed to overcome the
emotional discomfort of facing the unpleasant truths about oneself
with which an analysis confronts the analysand. In addition, there are
the burdens of frequent and inconvenient sessions, the expense of
time, effort, and money, and the embarrassment of being a "mental
patient." Some therapists judge a patient's motivation for treatment
to be insufficient for psychoanalysis if the prospective patient does
not manifest a wish to change. The more a therapist conceptualizes
pathology in terms of holding on to instinctual pleasures, and the
more, therefore, treatment is understood to help the patient to tame
and renounce his infantile aims, the more treatment will be conducted in an ambience devoid of those conventional aspects of an
ordinary social situation that could be interpreted as yearnings for
derivatives of these infantile strivings. Commonly, such concepts of
treatment generate an adversarial posture and require from the
patient a willingness to suffer uncommon frustration. It is thought
that only a painful dissatisfaction and concomitant wish to change
oneself will yield the requisite motivation to undergo and to work
through the displeasures attending analytic treatment.

The ambience becomes friendlier and more relaxed when the
therapist conceptualizes the treatment process less in terms of the
patient's having to effect a renunciation of neurotic pleasures and
more as providing an experience for the accretion of needed structure and strength. In a properly conducted therapy, the reigning
ambience allows the process of gaining strength to come about
without any conscious effort on the part of the patient. In this
respect, it resembles the processes of growth during development
that also proceed automatically in accord with the epigenetic pro-

gram if the proper conditions exist. It is therefore improper to demand a desire to "change" from a prospective patient. Individuals who have undergone analyses that are regarded as successful (by them and by their therapists) feel better and act better, but in some basic fundamentals they have not changed. They are the same people, with the same characteristic personalities, the same idiosyncratic constellation of likes and dislikes; the same basic ambitions, talents, and values; the same configuration of anxieties and depressions, though quantitatively ameliorated. The continuity of the self guarantees the continuity of basic patterns.

A patient's promise to change has no more meaning than a child's promise to grow an inch. Under the appropriate conditions it will happen, otherwise it will not. Extracting a promise to change implies a power that the patient does not have and knows he or she does not have. Such a demand to change is likely to make the patient feel either guilty or ashamed or both because of his or her presumed deficiency and inability. It is obvious that the prospective patient wants to change something and came in spite of inconvenience or shame about consulting a mental health professional. The desired change is most likely an unpleasant affect—a psychic pain, for example, anxiety, depression, shame, fear, guilt, disgust, horror, or the like. In a nutshell, the patient wants to feel better. No other motivation is needed for good analytic work.

Does this mean that patients do not achieve any real changes in psychotherapy?

A professional man in his mid-thirties came into analysis because he felt chronically anxious. In his dealings with colleagues and superiors he was timid to the point of feeling painfully shy at times. He experienced his marriage to a woman he had known since childhood as lacking joy and draining his energies because his wife had settled into a complaining passivity where she was unable to contribute much to their common family goals. During the analysis, his yearning for confirmation of his self—a mirror transference—was frequently disrupted, leading to transient depressed regressions when he experienced some unempathic comment by me as lacking the proper concern for his welfare. Associations led to memories of having been left alone to play with a younger sibling, for hours it seemed, and he recalled how he thought they had been forgotten. Working through his fear of abandonment as it manifested in the transference in innumerable forms led gradually to a significant reduction in his discomfort with himself: He became more cheerful, more self-confident, more assertive with his wife, friends, and professional contacts. The defenses that had protected him against the dangers of rejection, by keeping him isolated and uninvolved, faded into the background and no longer kept him from enthusiastically engaging in social intercourse. His wife also began an analysis and as a result, in conjunction with his greater availability to her, both finished her professional training and had a child.

This brief vignette does not touch on the many issues that were analyzed. But even this barest outline provides an overview that would make it difficult to argue that the analyses of these two people were not successful. Yet both people remained essentially and recognizably the same. No one would have thought that they had become different sorts of people, and only the most intimate of their friends would have noticed any changes at all. Still, the small changes that had occurred were of the greatest importance and account for turning depressed sterile lives into satisfyingly productive ones.

SUCCESS OR FAILURE?

Whether the patient and the therapist together will succeed in reaching the patient's goal depends on many factors and usually cannot be predicted with certainty. With luck, that is, barring any unforeseen and unforeseeable difficulties, and given a reasonably intact patient and a reasonably competent therapist, they should succeed, maybe, three out of four times: not such a bad percentage at all when compared with the results of the treatment of other serious chronic impairments that human beings fall heir to.

Why do some treatments fail? Assuming a well-analyzed and well-trained therapist, we often do not know the reasons for therapeutic failures. A number of explanations have been suggested.

Lack of Empathy

Among these explanations are the therapist's inability to be sufficiently empathic with the particular patient in question though he or she may be quite capable of good empathic contact with other patients.

Idiosyncratic Incompatibilities

Individuals—therapists as well as patients—have their own idiosyncratic qualities, and in the analytic situation these may clash rather than yield a therapeutic fit. Sometimes therapist and patient not only remind each other of their respective parents—the expected transferences and countertransferences—but sometimes, in actuality, the other person in the room does resemble very closely the remembered and dreaded archaic imago. In either case, the two parties may evoke in each other unacceptable affects associated with traumatic memories. Usually these transferences and countertransferences can be worked through. However, if the therapist does in fact closely resemble the early caregiver, working through becomes much more difficult and sometimes even problematic. The undogmatic analyst will usually recognize such an actual resemblance and, being alert to this danger, he or she avoids making an erroneous transference interpretation. Because so much depends on the fitting together of two individuals, the patient and the therapist, it is a good rule of thumb not to label a patient as unanalyzable unless there has been a trial of treatment with at least two and preferably three different therapists.

Excessive Damage

Finally, the patient may be too severely damaged psychologically, his or her self too fragile for the stresses and strains of a rigorous therapeutic process, and his or her ability to mobilize a minimum of basic trust too compromised.

TREATMENT PROCESS

Conceptually, one can distinguish two paths to strengthening the self. In actual clinical practice, both types of process often operate simultaneously on the arrested as well as on the distorted structures.

Via the Ambience

No self is totally free of areas where its development was arrested. Potentials of the self that are capable of being reactivated remain even when the ambience during development was by and large stimulating and facilitating. For a small number of patients, however, the accepting ambience of being in the presence of a respected person who is seriously, nonjudgmentally, and empathically interested in the patient's inner world may be the first such experience in their life. Treatment becomes the first occasion to be in a milieu that facilitates the healing of the self by allowing those aspects of the self which had been arrested in their development to resume developing. Thus, the selfs of such patients may finally recover somewhat from the early trauma resulting from faulty selfobject experiences. Still, there will remain scars and at least part of the pathologically heightened needs for distorted selfobject experiences.

Via the Disruption–Restoration Process

Frequently, the vulnerable self has been injured through faulty selfobject experiences, and the self has undergone traumatically induced distortions, leaving it crippled and malfunctioning in certain aspects.[3] Such distortions of the self secondary to injury appear to be more than arrested development, but they manifest as serious and deeper-going weakening of the self in conjunction with defensive structures. Archaic selfobject needs dominate in a weakened self and demand the experience of a total response. In contrast, mature selfobject needs can be satisfied by partial and measured responsiveness. Such injuries to the self are not repaired by a therapeutic ambience alone. Fortunately, there is a second and extremely important avenue for strengthening in psychotherapy the self weakened by structural malformation. This restoration of a strengthened self comes about via the disruption–restoration process that I spoke about earlier. The needs for fixated and defensively distorted archaic and primitive (and thus pathological) selfobject responses are re-

3. Kohut speaks about two kinds of structures that emerge in response to faulty selfobject experiences: defensive structures and compensatory structures (Kohut, 1977).

placed with age-appropriate needs for selfobject responses. I described this in overview as the step-wise replacement of archaic pathology with a selfobject response that one might label reciprocal empathic resonance. I will discuss this process now in some detail.

THE DISRUPTION–RESTORATION PROCESS

Resistance Analysis

The individual's always-present needs for selfobject responses emanate both from (1) residues of archaic needs modified by defenses, and (2) contemporaneous configurations. In the therapeutic situation, these ever-present selfobject needs tend to mobilize and manifest as more or less unconscious hopes or demands on the therapist. An accepting ambience will facilitate this mobilization, but even under the most propitious circumstances the fears carried forward from the past will interfere with the open expression of the mobilized needs. In other words, the patient resists the expression and even the awareness of these needs. An analytic interpretation of these resistances against the spontaneous emergence of these selfobject demands on the therapist facilitates mobilization of the selfobject transferences. Then the mobilized transferences will structure the relationship with the therapist in such a way that the therapist will be experienced as either performing or as refusing to perform the needed selfobject functions. Resistances protect against new injuries. Overcoming these resistances means that the injured self dares open itself up to a potential experience of being injured again.

In other words, the self entrusts itself to the therapist's capacity and willingness to perform the selfobject function. It is not easy to trust a stranger when past experience with the significant figures in one's life has usually been full of misunderstandings and ill-considered moralistic judgments. Will the therapist be competent and fair-minded? Will he or she really understand? The patient's self suspects that new disappointments and new injuries will occur again, as has happened before on numerous other occasions before coming into treatment.

In fact, the therapist inevitably will disappoint and fail to meet his or her own and the patient's expectations. But hope will not die easily, and it becomes part of the therapist's task to encourage these re-awakened yearnings by his or her professional commitment and an open attitude of being responsive to the patient's need for understanding. A cold rigidity during these early phases of resistance analysis can be like a killing frost, and a therapeutic process may not ever develop. For in essence, resistance is nothing but fear of being traumatically injured again. The decisive event of resistance analysis is the emergence of the patient's courage out of the experience of being accepted and empathically understood rather than being judged by the therapist. Such an accepting ambience facilitates the effectiveness of resistance interpretations, which otherwise fall on deaf ears whether they are correct or not. I believe this ambience to be more important than the exact verbal content of the resistance interpretations. The analytic situation beckons regression and mobilization of repressed and disavowed selfobject needs, while at the same time threatening traumatic disappointment. The therapist's calmly responsive strength facilitates the mobilization, while his nonjudgmental interpretations of the resistances diminish the fear of a repetition of the trauma. A vignette will illustrate:

A woman, a mental health professional, came thirty-five minutes late for her first appointment and announced that she did not really come for treatment but to have some things explained to her. I confess that I considered reminding her that I was seeing her as a therapist, not as an instructor, that I wished and had chosen to do analytic work with people who desired such services, and that I was not in the business of teaching or explaining psychotherapy in my office. As you can tell, I felt hurt, and I came close to revealing my injured self, which was demanding patient-like behavior from my prospective patient. But my momentary outrage passed as I began to listen and to hear a desperately fragile self open itself up ever so slightly to being injured again, while ostensibly surrounding itself with a barrage of denials of its needs. So I said very little, and very soon we made another appointment to which the patient came only twenty minutes late. I won't draw out this vignette. Suffice it to say that it did not take very long for a genuine treatment situation to evolve, which, however, could not be explicitly acknowledged by either one of us for a long time. Eventually, of course, the defensive behavior—personally, I don't like the term "resistance" because it has taken on some moral connotations of evil—could be interpreted explicitly. Had I actually needed appropriate patient-like behavior on that first day in order to properly feel myself a therapist, I wonder if I would have found this patient untreatable. Or perhaps I would have thought her a borderline.

Transference Mobilization

The second step in the disruption–restoration process is the *spontaneous mobilization of the patient's selfobject transferences.* I wish to stress that patients are in constant conflict. The conflict is between the constant need for selfobject responses, on the one hand, and the fear of the self's being injured, on the other hand. Most of the time, the fears are dominant and they thwart movement toward establishing selfobject relationships that can become self-sustaining selfobject experiences. Consequently, the patients coming into treatment are usually starved for needed selfobject responses. When the therapeutic ambience, in combination with resistance analysis, creates an experience of relatively greater safety for the patient, then the balance between need and fear shifts, the ever-present hope is encouraged, and the rising expectation that the selfobject needs will be heard and understood leads to an intensification of these needs, which then override the fear. Though at first revealed only hesitantly, the most important of the patient's expectations of the therapist is to be understood. The therapist's empathic understanding brings about a general mobilization and revival of archaic, repressed, and disavowed selfobject needs that determine the expectations focused on the therapist and thus shape the selfobject transference: a mutual experience of well-being testifies that a harmonious transference has emerged.

Transference Disruption

The third step in the process ensues when the spontaneously established sustaining selfobject *transference is disrupted.* This transference disruption comes about just as spontaneously as the establishment of the transference, and it occurs inevitably because the therapist is bound to "fail" in maintaining a total and perfect empathic "in tuneness" with the patient. At some point, the patient suddenly feels outraged, often thinking that the therapist seems more interested in his or her own agenda—which is making a correct interpretation—than in the patient's burning concern at that moment—which is to be compassionately understood. And, indeed, the chances are that the patient's perceptions are correct and not a distortion. For at that moment the patient does not really wish to be scrutinized and analyzed and hear an interpretation, but wants to experience the therapist's empathy. Yet, to point this out would be just another instance of the same misunderstanding and widen the breach. Before such an interpretation can usefully be made, therefore, the therapist must acknowledge the patient's perception of the therapist's "failure" as real, regardless of whether it is the result of the patient's distortion or not. The patient's experience must be validated before it can be usefully interpreted.

Transference Regressions

Disruptions of the selfobject transference cause a temporary regression to previous, more archaic modes of relationship, which then may be characterized by defensively distorted and exaggerated demands on the therapist or by defensively motivated distancing and withdrawal and sometimes also by acting out. Please note that distorted perceptions of the therapist by the patient are not the cause of the disruption, but may be the result. Also note that defensiveness here does not mean defense against instinctual intrusion; on the contrary, the temporary regression of the self to a state of lessened cohesion in this case is often accompanied by some disintegration of the self with the emergence of distorted fragments of sexuality and aggression, for example, perversions and other forms of acting out.

The defensive nature of these more archaic modes of relating, that is, the detachment, or the sexualization, or the aggressivization, is evident from their being used in the defense of the remaining self-structure. The disappointing selfobject may be held at a safer distance by the often obnoxious quality of these defensively used manifestations of disintegration, or it may be brought closer by the evident neediness. Either way, the self, though in pain and need and at reduced functional capacity, tries to marshal whatever resources, including the products of its own disintegration, to influence the carrier of the selfobject function into a posture of supplying the need.

It is the archaic, distorted, and imperative nature of the revived selfobject need that often makes it, in fact, counterproductive in ordinary social intercourse. In the therapy, however, at least ideally, the therapist by virtue of his or her empathy and theoretical orientation, can recognize the legitimate selfobject needs underlying their distorted and archaic manifestations, manifestations that he or she experiences often with some discomfort as well.

Transference Restoration

This then leads to the fourth step, the *restoration of the self-object transference through proper interpretation* of the transference disruption. The therapist explains and interprets to the patient the sequence of events that led to the disruption. This requires tact, an empathic understanding of how the patient experienced and thought about the disruption, and, last but not least, how it was experienced and understood by the therapist.

Because he is introspectively in contact with his own inner psychic reality and empathically attuned to his patient's different reality and suffering, the analyst is in a good position to discern what actions committed or omitted may have precipitated the present impasse. Perhaps he will come to the recognition that the disruption is due to a break in correctly sensing each other's inner experiences: not only an erroneous attunement of the analyst to the patient's needs but also an equally erroneous reading of the analyst's intentions on part of the patient, the latter often as a result of transference of archaic fears and expectations. The therapist therefore will explore for clues that will explain the disruption and grope for ways of communicating his understanding, that is, conveying his insight to the patient via interpretation. This exploratory and explaining effort of the analyst is experienced by the patient as evidence of his concerns being taken seriously. For both, but especially for the analysand, this is an experience of his own efficacy in eliciting an attuned response, of having made a dent, of being somebody, a confirmed self. Healing experiences in psychoanalytic treatment require (1) a sense of being understood by the other and (2) a sense of one's own efficacy regarding the other. We cannot, with our present state of knowledge in psychoanalytic psychology, say much about the relative contribution of the various types of mirroring, idealizing, or alter-ego selfobject experiences nor of the experience of efficacy to the cohesion of the self. But it seems clear that all of them are essential requirements for the emergence of a strong self. One could conceptualize the need for efficacy pleasure as a variety of a needed mirroring experience. However, in view of its extra-analytic validation by mother-infant observations involving responses from a non-living object, I think it best to conceive the need for efficacy experiences as a separate kind of need (cf. pp. 60-62).

Conceptually, it is important to point out that the disruptions, like the preceding harmonious selfobject transference, are not new experiences with a new object. Rather, what is new is that the therapist does not respond in the manner of an ordinary social situation, but responds by explaining and interpreting on the basis of an empathically informed understanding. More specifically, although the therapist's initial posture may have been experienced by the patient as if the therapist were a figure from the past—and, indeed, the therapist for his or her own reasons does act very often as if he or she were a parent or other closely related individual—the therapist also acts differently by taking an emotional distance, that is, by accepting the patient's experience without insisting that his or her own experience be the measure of all things. Even the therapist's well-thought out explanations are subject to correction by the patient. Such explanations given within an accepting ambience based on the therapist's empathic attunement to the patient are not gratifications of a need—neither of a selfobject need nor of an instinctual wish or need—except for the need to be understood. By again feeling understood, the empathic flow between therapist and patient is restored.

A successful disruption-restoration process restores the mutual reciprocal empathic flow between patient and therapist. One commonly observes that the restored empathic bond is stronger and less vulnerable to repeated disruptions. However, disruptions will still occur, albeit less frequently and less intensely loaded with affect, when the inevitable disjunctions in the reciprocal empathic flow recur. Yet unmistakably, the patient's self grows stronger and its selfobject needs are gradually transformed into more mature, age-appropriate modes. The patient's extra-analytic functioning improves, as does the quality and the satisfactions derived from extra-analytic relationships.

It is easy to explain that intra-analytically the self's strength is restored with the resumption of the empathic bond because the analyst again is available as a provider of sustaining selfobject experiences. But the observation of a self stronger than before the disruption and, particularly, a self gaining new strength outside the analytic situation requires the assumption that the disruption-restoration experience is equivalent to a learning experience that has resulted in a rearranged or reorganized self structure. Apparently, the regression brought about by the analytic process is a precondition for this reorganization. The patient exercises some of the functions of the self that are involved in scanning, perceiving, and responding to a selfobject matrix, perhaps for the first time since infancy and childhood. These functions can now be exercised in the analytic situation because of the ambience of safety created by the analytic therapist. Exercising these functions strengthens them the way muscles are strengthened by use.

The mutual reciprocal empathic therapeutic dialogue is such an exercise, and it is fundamentally different from pretherapeutic dialogues with family and friends. One difference is the therapeutic regression, which allows the involvement of formerly deeply hidden and unconscious aspects of functions. The other difference is the consistent attitude of empathic understanding by the analytic therapist. The patient's experience of safety and trust gradually extinguishes the almost automatically reflexive defensive maneuvers, thereby facilitating experimentation with new modes of perceiving and responding. The experimental modes that have worked in the therapeutic situation can then be tried outside this sphere of relative safety, where the patient discovers, to his or her surprise, that benign selfobject experiences can also occur outside the therapeutic relationship. The responsiveness of extratherapeutic selfobjects further strengthens the self. The pretherapy vicious cycle of faulty responses leading to fragmentation, leading to more faulty responses has been replaced by a cycle of appropriate responsiveness leading to greater cohesion, leading to better functioning. It is a learning process that depends not on information supplied by interpretation but on an experience that can be explained.

The Mutative Character of
Disruption–Restoration Experiences

But, one may ask, how does an experience become mutative, that is, how does the experience change the self in such a way that it is stronger after the mutative experience than before? Let us recall briefly that the very emergence of the self depends on appropriate selfobject experiences, among which the mirroring selfobject experience is an essential component. To paraphrase this mirroring experience one might say that one exists as a self because a significant someone knows and addresses us as a peson, a self. This significant someone has been designated by self psychology as a selfobject, and its function in evoking the self experience in the subject has been called a selfobject experience. I have also mentioned that regardless of presenting symptoms or behavior—whether anxious, hostile or depressed, whether arrogant or pleasing, compliant or rebelliously acting out—there exists, ubiquitously, in the patient a feeling of badness of the self. It is a more or less unconscious but apparently unshakable conviction of one's self (and person) being faulty and unacceptable in some fundamental way that already became part of the self's very structure when it was constituted and emerged as a self. The baby's natural and blissful experience of itself in its grandiose glory was spoiled almost from the start by a pathogenic mirroring selfobject experience: the selfobject acted or functioned as if the baby was experienced by the selfobject as bad. Perhaps this represents the selfobject's psychopathology, or perhaps it reflects unfortunate circumstances that skewed the selfobject experience and warped the emerging self.

In the analytic situation when, after much analytic work, the layers of defenses, symptoms, and behavior have been laid bare for both analyst and analysand to see, there then remains the patient's core conviction of essential badness. No words, no verbal interpretation alone can correct this depressive core. Even the explicit reassurance by an empathic analyst during an intense transference relationship will not remedy any more effectively than the compassion of friends and family. Neither empathy nor love cures.

I have described the therapeutic process that culminates in disruption-restoration sequences. Under certain conditions such a disruption-restoration experience may reach the depressed core of the self and change it by rearranging its constituents. To achieve such a desired outcome there have to be (1) a regression that is deep enough to loosen the self's structure without endangering its cohesion and boundaries, and (2) an analyst who not only is able to skillfully manage the disruption-restoration process but who, in addition, knows with sincere conviction that, indeed, the analysand is not bad but human, with inevitable frailties and limitations. This analyst cannot help but create a selfobject experience for the analysand that is different than the one with the original selfobjects; that is, the self that emerges from the therapeutic regression will have as part of its constitutive experience the conviction of essential goodness. Over time and many disruptions and restorations, this patient will gradually gain a new perspective on his person and self that will imbue him with the strength to cope with the human condition.

REGRESSIONS

The analytic disruption–restoration process just outlined is predicated, among other factors, on the self being sufficiently strong to withstand the stress of the emotional upheaval, and, especially, the painful disruptions of the transference, without undue regression or total and perhaps irreversible fragmentation of the self.

Therapeutic Regressions

In the psychoanalytic situation, especially, a regressive process in the patient is facilitated. The basic rule to say everything that comes to mind, thereby requiring the patient to relinquish some control over his or her speech, imposes tension, as does the frustration evoked by not being responded to in a normal social manner. In addition, the patient is in a supine position and unable to see the therapist, who is sitting behind him or her. As a patient regresses, the process has a loosening effect on the structure and boundaries of the self, with a further mobilization of the residuals of long repressed or disavowed selfobject needs. These changes brought about by the regressive pull of the therapeutic situation facilitate the analytic work, because the mobilized archaic structures thus can become the core of the selfobject transferences. The regression also interferes with learned logico-cognitive thought-processing and lessens the firmness of the self's boundaries, making them more permeable to empathic communications. Usually, such a mild regression engendered by the analytic situation has no deleterious consequences and makes the therapeutic process possible.

Severe Regressions

In some people, however, the fragile structure of the self makes the self vulnerable to uncontrolled regression. That is, there is a danger that the regressive process, once initiated, cannot be satisfactorily controlled and may progress to a psychotic-like state. In most people with such vulnerable selfs, defenses have been erected during development to protect the self against these dangerous regressions. These defenses take various forms; among them, schizoid mechanisms, paranoid mechanisms, and the rigidities of certain obsessive-compulsive preoccupations have been described in great detail in the psychotherapeutic and psychoanalytic literature.

These defenses serve to keep the person relatively isolated and away from noxious relationships that might lead to traumatic self-object experiences. The diagnosis of borderline state is often applied to such people. People with such vulnerable selfs manifest in the analytic situation the symptoms associated with these defenses. Symptoms of untoward regressions should alert the therapist to take steps to slow the regressive process until the self has gained sufficient strength to maintain control over its own state of organization. Among the various interventions in the therapist's armamentarium are medications (anti-depressants, anxiolytics), changing the frequency of sessions (some respond to a reduction in frequency, others to an increase), changing from the use of the couch to face-to-face treatment, and focusing away from the exploration of fantasy to a more reality-directed concern.

Treatability

Psychological treatment facilitates regression and increases the vulnerability of the self to react to noxious stimuli with decreased cohesion, increased permeability of boundaries, and mobilization of repressed or split-off affects. The capacity to regress, therefore, is a necessary precondition for making repressed and split-off parts of the self accessible to the interactive therapeutic process. On the other hand, excessive regression may mean dangerous degrees of loss of cohesion, that is, fragmentation, and, similarly dangerous degrees of losing boundaries. Therefore, it is necessary to evaluate the regressive potential early in the assessment of patients for psychoanalytic treatment. The conventional classification into psychoses, borderline states, and personality disorders is not always a reliable guide, nor does a diagnosis of a classical psychoneurotic syndrome rule out the possibility of untoward regressions. The criteria of the Diagnostic and Statistical Manual of the American Psychiatric Association (DSM-III-R) allow one to classify into appropriate categories after one has made a judgment regarding the regressive state and potential. How does one arrive at that judgment?

The most important information comes from an accurate history, since in almost all cases the danger of excessive regression is signaled by a history of prior occurrences of such regressive episodes. On the positive side, a history of a prospective analysand's having withstood severely traumatic events associated with intense states of fear, anger, or depression without signs of serious loss of self-control in behavior or serious disturbances in usually solid interpersonal relationships bodes well for also withstanding the rigors of a psychoanalytic endeavor without undue consequences. To gather this information takes time and mutual trust. The therapeutic undertaking must proceed with a certain tentativeness while watching how the therapeutic regression is developing. The decision to treat someone psychotherapeutically, regardless whether the mode of treatment is supportive, relationship therapy or psychoanalysis, is not a one-time act but emerges as an ongoing process of observation and reevaluation. Although, perhaps, psychotic patients regress more easily or deeply than borderline patients and neurotic patients, and personality disorders usually are less inclined to undergo severe regressions, this is not at all a reliable guide. Diagnostic assessment and treatment decisions are not safely made before treatment starts but grow out of the treatment process itself. Patients who have never achieved a cohesive self are most vulnerable to excessive regressions and not suitable for regression-inducing treatment modalities. Patients with a history of psychosis, particularly schizophrenia and severe dysthymic disorders usually ought to be managed with the aid of psychopharmaceuticals.

What About the Psychoneuroses?

Injured selfs that nevertheless achieved a measure of cohesion such as we find in the narcissistic personality disorders and in the narcissistic behavior disorders are the prime candidates for psychotherapy. What about the psychoneuroses? In my experience, pure symptom neurosis has become a rarity, and the patients with whom I have had the privilege of working during the last years all suffered from primary selfobject relations pathology. Many also suffered from a variety of neurotic sexual pathology derived from pathological oedipal complexes, but in each case the oedipal pathology was the result of faulty responses by the oedipal selfobjects of childhood. Psychoneurosis thus seems to be a particular variety of selfobject pathology and is treated as such.[4]

FURTHER COMMENTS ON TREATMENT AMBIENCE

I have designated the experience of the psychotherapeutic situation and process the psychoanalytic ambience (Wolf, 1976a). The very possibility of the therapeutic process occurring and progressing toward increased strength of the self concomitant with improved comprehension of the self by the self is contingent on the establishment and maintenance of an analytic ambience of respect, acceptance, and understanding. It is important to remember that the psychoanalytic process explores experiences, not absolute truth.

A variety of descriptive terms are in common usage, and they can be paired, for example, tense versus relaxed, warm versus cold, accepting versus rejecting, critical versus nonjudgmental, reasoned versus dogmatic, misunderstanding versus understanding, friendly versus hostile, cooperative versus adversarial, interested versus indifferent, and so forth. Different people probably would not agree in their assessment of a particular ambience, especially if they were judging as nonparticipant observers—attempting to be objective from the outside, so to speak. It seems, similarly, that each of the two participants in an analytic situation and process often experience a totally different ambience.

---

4. Self psychology is frequently misunderstood to be dismissing all sexuality as mere disintegration products. To be sure, pathological and neurotic sexuality are conceptualized as deriving from faulty selfobject experiences which have fragmented the self and yielded disintegration products that have been organized into neurotic symptoms or sexualized behavior. But even the healthy single individual with a firmly cohesive self must be seen as incomplete in the larger context of a life, and normally will be striving to complete himself or herself by sexual union with an individual of the opposite sex.

Patients also differ widely in their experience of the therapeutic ambience. What one patient might perceive as warm and friendly might be experienced by another as cold and distant. In the analytic situation one man's meat truly is another man's poison. The analytic ambience as experienced by the patient determines to a large extent whether the analytic process will stalemate and derail or whether it will go forward.

Transference Interpretation

Kohut (1971, p. 291, 291*n*.) stresses, like Freud, the great importance of avoiding premature interpretations of the transference. According to Kohut, the analyst should not interfere (either by premature interpretations or by other means) with the spontaneous mobilization of the transference wishes. The interpretive work concerning the transference should begin only at the point when, because of nonfulfillment of the transference wishes, the patient's cooperation ceases, that is, when the transference has become a resistance. Interpretative references to the transference, especially early in the course of the analysis, will be correctly understood by the patient as prohibitions. No matter how friendly and kindly the analyst expresses himself, the analysand will hear him say: "Don't be that way—it's unrealistic, childish!" or the like.

On the other hand, Kohut speaks of three common resistances surrounding the transference as it is being established, and he does advocate their early interpretation. Three fears predominate during this initial analytic phase, and they all relate to dangers associated with the analytic process. Kohut (1971, p. 88) mentions the patient's fear of regression, his apprehension vis-à-vis a difficult task, and his fear of the extinction of his personality by the deep wish to merge with and into the idealized object. Kohut suggests that the analyst acknowledge the presence of all these resistances and define them to the patient with friendly understanding, but he need do nothing further to provide reassurance. In a more general vein, analysts must realize that there are indeed moments in an analysis when even the most cogent and correct interpretation about any detail of the patient's personality is out of place and, for instance, unacceptable to the patient who seeks a comprehensive response to a recent important event in his or her life (Kohut, 1971, p. 121).

Freud told us that, like government, we are engaged in an impossible profession. Perhaps that is true if our aim is to change us and make the world a reasonable place. Instead, we may have to be satisfied with gaining a few increments of sense and strength with which to push back the encroachments of unreason. We have not got much to show for our efforts, except that our patients lead fuller, more creative, and more satisfying lives. And that is a lot.

. 10 .

SELFOBJECT TRANSFERENCES

Clinical transferences are the manifestations in the clinical analytic situation of distorted archaic needs and the defenses against them that were acquired during childhood in interaction with the earliest selfobjects.

However, it is easy to forget that there is always also a trigger in the current here-and-now situation that pulls the memories and defenses of the archaic past into the present situation as transference. Sometimes the analyst may behave in such a way as to appear totally unreasonable or hostile or seductive or unacceptable in some other way to the analysand. Intense reactions, for example, in the defense of remaining self structure, may be provoked by such behavior in the current situation without necessarily containing any significant aspects of transference from the past.

TYPES

Merger Transference

Merger transference is the re-establishment in the analytic situation of an experience of identity with the (self)object of early development through an extension of the self to include the (selfobject)analyst in it. It manifests by an expectation that the analyst not be a center of initiative (i.e., an agent, in Kohut's phrase), but that he be totally subject to the patient's initiative, for example, like the patient's limbs. Sometimes the patient expects the analyst to be so attuned to his or her needs and thoughts that he know them without being told by the patient. Sometimes the merger transference manifests first by the defenses against it, that is, by an excessive need to remain at an apparent distance from the selfobject, for example, in schizophrenic-like isolation or in schizoid or paranoid character armor. The defense is necessary to protect against the overwhelming trauma that would be experienced if the needed merger with the selfobject should miscarry because of the selfobject's reluctance to become enmeshed and be controlled.

It is often very difficult to discern what were the root causes for the self's vulnerability during a particular individual's development. Was it the parent's fear of enmeshment with the infant that came first, or was it the infant's need to withdraw in order to avoid traumatic affects? Was the latter need a reaction to perceiving or misperceiving parental intrusiveness, or was it an inborn lethargic temperament? Other constellations of infant–caregiver interactions and associated selfobject experiences may have left their imprint on the developing self. One hopes that the transference experience with the analyst will yield clues that the analyst can recognize as developmental re-experiences that are interpretable.

Mirror Transference

Unfortunately, the term "mirror transference" was used by Kohut in two ways: (1) as a generic term for several types of transferences that affirm the self—that is, the mirror, merger and alter-ego transferences—and (2) mirror transference proper, in contradistinction to the idealizing transference. This has led to a certain confusion and I am restricting myself to using the term only in the second sense. The mirror transference proper refers to the re-establishment of an early need for acceptance and confirmation of the self by the selfobject. It manifests as demands on the analyst (or defenses against such demands) to confirm the patient's self by recognizing, admiring, or praising the patient.

Alter-ego Transference

Alter-ego transference is the re-experience of an early need that peaks during latency—a need to see and understand another who is like oneself, as well as to be seen and be understood by someone like oneself. Kohut initially classified the alter-ego transference as one of the generic type of mirror transferences, but later emphasized it as a separate type of transference. It manifests as a need, in general, to be like the analyst in appearance, manner, outlook, and opinion. Developmentally, the alter-ego relationship is associated with the fantasy of an imaginary playmate and is important in the acquisition of skills and competences.

Idealizing Transference

Idealizing transference is the re-establishment of the need for an experience of merging with a calm, strong, wise, and good selfobject. It may manifest as the more or less disguised admiration of the analyst, his or her character and values, or by defenses against this transference, such as prolonged and bitter depreciation of the analyst.

Transference of Creativity

Transference of creativity is Kohut's (1976) term for the transient need of certain creative personalities for an experience of merger with a selfobject while engaged in the most taxing creative tasks. An example might be Freud's need for Fliess during the writing of *The Interpretation of Dreams* (1900).

Adversarial Transference

The adversarial transference is the need to experience a supportive yet oppositional selfobject relationship, an ally–antagonist selfobject experience (cf. Wolf, 1980c, pp. 125–126). The two-year-old who responds to all communications with "No" is acting out a need to experience himself or herself as autonomous and to have his or her autonomy responsively accepted.

TECHNICAL ASPECTS OF MIRRORING

A clinical vignette (Kohut, 1971) will illustrate.

Miss F would become violently angry and accuse the analyst of undermining and wrecking the analysis if the analyst's interpretation went a single step beyond what she had actually told him, even if what the analyst added was already known to her. Her intolerance of hearing from the analyst anything that she already knew speaks against her behavior being a resistance to making the unconscious conscious. She was not afraid of hearing something that she did not want to know or of hearing again something she already knew. It was not a matter of knowing at all. She could tolerate knowledge but could not tolerate the position of the analyst as a center of initiative. Her assertive behavior directed toward the analyst suggests a claim that the analyst must be completely submissive to her own thinking, that he must relinquish any initiative of his own, and that he devote himself to nothing but the acceptance and affirmation of whatever aspect of herself she was presenting to him. She expected the analyst to be, in fact, an extension of her own self.

"His Majesty the Baby"

A claim such as Miss F's is reminiscent of an absolute yet insecure monarch's attitude toward his subjects. The complementary attitude that these lowly subjects are expected to have toward their exalted monarch brings to mind Freud's felicitous phrase "His Majesty the Baby," by which he meant the idealizing attitude of affectionate parents toward their small children, and which he recognized as a revival and reproduction of their own archaic narcissism (Freud, 1914, p. 90-91). One might say that the mirror transference is the re-enactment of the archaic claims of "His Majesty the Baby" in the here-and-now of the analytic situation. Because these archaic claims are universal and ubiquitous—Freud connected them to the primary narcissism of children (Freud, 1914, p. 90)—they can be conceptualized as a direct expression of infantile narcissism. In self-psychological terms, these demands are recognized as the imperative need of any child for confirmation. The designations "narcissistic" or "grandiose" are external rather than empathic judgments about the self-object experience and often convey a disdainful attitude.

Archaic or Contemporaneous Needs?

We are left with a number of questions that are important for the conduct of an analysis. Have these archaic and infantile demands remained especially prominent in this patient? And why is this patient seeking a compliant response from the analyst so insistently now? Usually such demands are not verbalized explicitly, but enacted in the transference as expectations. Eventually, however, with a diminution of fears, defenses, and resistances, patients may well verbalize the full extent of their expectations from the analyst and of their outraged disappointments at the analyst's failure to comply.[1] These expectations are then seen to be derived not only from current pressures, but also from earlier experiences that did not reach a satisfactory conclusion and left a residue in the form of defects or distortions of the self.

Fear of Regression

Transference-like expectations and fears are ubiquitous in daily life, and all actions are influenced to a degree by the hopes carried forward from the archaic past. The special urgency and even peremptory power of transference within the psychoanalytic situation is the result of the regression that is facilitated by both the structure of the analytic situation and the ambience of a properly conducted analysis. Although the regression-enhanced transference makes interpretation and working-through possible, the patient's fear of the regressive pull of the analytic situation makes for powerful resistances, particularly early in the analytic process. Patients fear regressing to earlier, more archaic, and therefore more fragile self states. They shamefully dislike experiencing themselves as infantile in their demandingness and hate to experience the utter frustration and helplessness that come with not being responded to fully. But worse even than shame and rage, that is, worse than experiencing grandiosity and helplessness, is the panicky experience of the fragility of a self that is not affirmed and thus threatened with fragmentation and dissolution. It is not only the regression that threatens self cohesion, but for vulnerable patients, it is also the relative scarcity of selfobject responses in the analytic situation when compared with

---

1. Anyone who has worked within the self-psychological frame has experienced these outbreaks of rage. The criticism that the empathic stance of self psychologists leads to collusions that avoid dealing with hostility demonstrates the critic's unfamiliarity with actual self-psychological practice.

the average social milieu. Humiliation threatens to turn into mortification, into the deadly loss of self. On occasion, though rarely, a borderline patient's defenses against regression give way to a psychotic-like debacle, characterized by the loss of self structure with a return to an earlier psychological state of primitively organized and frequently deformed psychic structure. We can define the function of the selfobject as providing those experiences for the self that evoke and maintain the self's cohesion, that is, the mirroring, idealizing, and alter-ego experiences. Absent or faulty selfobject experiences inevitably are followed by impairment or loss of self structure.

Transference in the Service of Defense

Regression and the frustrations of relative abstinence, therefore, threaten the self in the analytic situation and mobilize powerful defenses that find expression in the relationship to the analyst—the transference. On the other hand, the analyst, by virtue of his implied promise of being a healer, by his reputation for knowledge and skill, and, last but certainly not least, by his personality, may well tend to encourage the patient's expectations for relief from suffering. Old repressed and disavowed longings for closeness to a source of selfobject responses are re-awakened and contribute to a mobilization of the analysand's selfobject needs. Thus, in essence, underneath the shell of arrogance, the mirror transference is the imperative demand on the analyst to provide an affirmative experience for the child, to soothe and strengthen the child's self and to keep it from regressing into a state of self dissolution—that is, into the early primitive psychological state from which a self had first emerged. Most analyses do not reach the deepest levels of regression, where the mirror transference manifests in its archaic essence, nor need most analyses reach that deeply into the core of the psyche. A satisfactory working-through process can be activated without first having regressed to the level of total fragmentation and disorganization.

But why is the affirmation of the child's archaic self by its parental selfobjects or of the regressed patient's reactivated and distorted infantile self by the therapist so necessary for the cohesion of the self? Why is the "good mother" one who concurs with her baby in the child's illusion of greatness, and why is the parent who debunks the child's grandiose pretensions thereby laying the groundwork for later psychopathology (cf. Wolf, 1985)? And why is it necessary for the analyst to affirm the patient—not by approval but by accepting and attempting to understand his or her thoughts, feelings, and behavior—before the analytic and interpretive work can proceed? An understanding of the fundamentals of the development of self–selfobject experiences will illuminate these phenomena.

Developmental Considerations

The need for selfobject responses is not confined to the archaic selfobjects that are the normal requirements of the early years. Selfobject responses in a variety of forms are needed throughout the life span. Indeed, the need for selfobject responses is always present, waxing and waning with the ups and downs of the strength and vulnerability of the self. At one end of the spectrum, the strong, healthy, and mature self still requires some mirroring affirmation even in a nourishingly stimulating environment that is free of noxious stresses; at the other end, the fragile or regressed or otherwise vulnerable self desperately needs the mirroring function exercised by a selfobject matrix to maintain some semblance of self cohesion, even when its fragility has activated powerful defenses—such as schizoid withdrawal or paranoid hostility—that frustrate and defeat the yearning for selfobject responses. Similarly, experiences with idealized selfobjects and alter-ego self objects are also needed over a lifetime. As the individual grows and matures from birth to death, the original archaic form of the selfobject needs of infancy gradually change into other forms of selfobject needs that are appropriate to the level of maturity reached. The developmental line of selfobject relations represents one way to conceptualize the changing requirements for selfobject experiences (Wolf, 1980c). But much remains to be done here also:

> . . . we need investigations of the special selfobject needs of adolescents and the elderly, for example, along with investigations of the selfobject needs that accompany specific life tasks including those shifts to a new cultural milieu that deprive a person of his "cultural selfobjects," during his mature years or when he has to deal with a debilitating illness, or the confrontation with death. (Kohut, 1984, p. 194)

SELFOBJECT TRANSFERENCES   131

The terminological shift from "narcissistic" transferences to "selfobject" transferences has still another significance. Although Kohut initially defined the need for mirroring as related to the reactivation of the archaic infantile grandiose self—and this is still true for the early years of childhood and for selfs in a state of relatively deep regression—we can define the need for mirroring now more generally as the universal need of any self to be affirmed as significant. Ideally, perhaps, one could wish for a self so strong, healthy, and cohesive as to have no need for selfobject experiences of any kind. Clinically, however, one cannot expect to come upon a self that needs neither the responses of a mirroring selfobject nor the availability of an idealizable selfobject.

THE USE AND MISUSE OF MIRRORING

Substitute for Previous Deprivation

The term "mirroring" is sometimes misused to designate a kind of supportive-sympathetic clinical activity that, mistakenly, is thought to be of help to patients whose self disorders manifest as a mirroring selfobject transference, such as a demand to be recognized, approved, or admired. A history of insufficient mirroring responses from the selfobjects of childhood serves as the rationale for being kind and gratifying, to substitute in the here-and-now for the deprivation the patient suffered in early development. Involved in this practice of "mirroring" is the hypothesis that the current misery follows directly from early analogous deprivations and that by providing a "corrective emotional experience" in the here-and-now the deficit can be repaired or at least filled in.

Empathy: Data or Deeds?

Parenthetically, one might also add that a misreading of Kohut's definition of empathy is involved. This misreading misconstrues empathy to be some sort of activity to influence the patient. According to Kohut, however, to be empathic means to be listening and perceiving in a certain way so as to grasp some aspects of the patient's inner experience. It is a method for the collection of psycho-analytic data. To be empathic does not mean to be doing something good for the patient. Indeed, the knowledge gained by being empathic can be used for or against the patient's benefit. To be sure, to sense that another human being does understand one and does have some inkling of what one is experiencing is very supportive to the structure of one's self and to one's experience of selfhood, and it is very enhancing to one's self-esteem. This is so even when the other person's intentions are inimical and the empathically gained knowledge is used destructively. The essence of a certain kind of salesmanship (or advertising) is exactly the salesman's empathic "in tuneness" with the customer's needs and wishes, and the ability to sell on the basis of making the customer feel that his needs and desires are understood, regardless of whether the sold product is really needed or perhaps even harmful.

Optimal Responsiveness

Sometimes patients can be helped to feel better, temporarily, by the therapist's approval, whether or not he or she really grasps the patient's inner experience. Approval may erroneously be experienced as empathy. Other patients sometimes find advice from the therapist quite useful. Except for some very regressed patients during certain traumatic and cohesion-threatening life crises, however, such active approbationary or advisory activity on the part of the therapist is not indicated and may do harm to the unfolding analytic process. To provide advice or approval when that is not needed creates an illusion of the therapist's wisdom and omnipotence against a background of the patient's incompetence. Patients may desire this during moments of an intense idealizing transference, but the patient's real need is to be understood and calls for interpretation rather than enactment. The misunderstanding may derive from the historical development of analytic technique. Classical analytic abstinence was indeed relatively nonempathic and nonresponsive, and Kohut's emphasis on an empathic stance was a reaction to the often fragmenting effects of excessive technical abstinence. Kohut's call for optimal frustration, however, recognized the limits of sympathy and kindness. Bacal (1985) usefully defines a balanced approach of "optimal responsiveness" ". . . as the responsivity of the analyst which is therapeutically relevant, at that moment, to his particular patient and his illness (p. 202)."

Therapeutic Ambience

Furthermore, the analytic work with analyzable disorders of the self should not be jeopardized by confusing the therapeutic regression brought about by the analytic process with pathological fixations or regressions rooted in an severely damaged self or resulting from overwhelming traumatic events in the patient's life, whether current or past. A desirable level of therapeutic regression results in the mobilization and reactivation of repressed and disavowed archaic selfobject needs that should be responded to by interpretation within an accepting analytic ambience (Wolf, 1976a). Let me restate with emphasis: "The analyst does not actively soothe; he interprets the analysand's yearning to be soothed. The analyst does not actively mirror; he interprets the need for confirming responses. The analyst does not actively admire or approve grandiose expectations; he explains their role in the psychic economy. The analyst does not fall into passive silence; he explains why his interventions are felt to be intrusive. Of course, the analyst's mere presence, or the fact that he talks, or, especially, the fact that he understands, all have soothing and self-confirming effects on the patient, *and they are so interpreted*" (Goldberg, 1978, pp. 447-48). Let me clarify, however, that an accepting analytic ambience, the *sine qua non* for making interpretations effective, can be experienced as strengthening to the structural integrity of the self. In some patients this strengthening experience may be needed for months or years before the verbally explicit interpretation can be added to or substituted for the message implicit in the analysand's experience of being attentively listened to and understood.

Genetic Ambience: Grandiose Illusions

It is different during infancy when children do need to be "mirrored", that is "to be looked upon with joy and basic approval by a delighted parental selfobject" (Kohut, 1984, p. 143). Indeed, one may say that parent and child enter into a conspiracy of illusion in which both seem to believe and tell each other that they are perfect. Such illusions of unique and blissfully superlative excellence are not only common but apparently a necessary experience in the developmental history of firm and cohesive selfs. Usually such an illusory overvaluation is willingly entered into by both infant and parent. The mother who refuses to enter into this conspiracy of illusion with her child—that is, the parent whose blinders exclude all vision except that of the "real world"—and who therefore confronts the child with the debunking reality of the child's smallness, weakness, or its innumerable other shortcomings will crush the developing self and surely plant the seeds for future self disorder.

But the analytic therapist is ill-advised when he believes he can repair the damage to the child's self by substituting an illusion in the here-and-now of the analytic situation for the missing illusions of infancy and childhood. Interpretation—based on empathic understanding of the state of the self and on its history—of the understandable needs and wishes for illusory reassurances can strengthen the self and allow it to give up defenses against needed selfobject closeness. The therapist accepts the patient's "outrageous" selfobject demand matter-of-factly as a naturally occurring expression of the need to strengthen the self through enhanced selfobject responsiveness. The therapist tries empathically to understand, and attempts to explain and interpret, but avoids gratification of archaic demands in order to keep the analytic process moving. If the therapist, instead of creating an ambience of acceptance, attempts to create an illusion of approbation and gratification, the patient will quickly discover the hollowness of the therapist's posture and feel betrayed. This may well derail the analytic as well as the therapeutic process.

Corrective Emotional Experience

"Mirroring" thus is not an appropriate activity in the usual analytic treatment process with analyzable disorders of the self. However, creating the proper ambience for (1) the mobilization of demands for "mirroring," and (2) the free expression of these demands is the responsibility of the analyst, as is their timely and tactful interpretation (Wolf, 1976a). As already noted, this facilitating ambience has sometimes been confused with what Alexander termed a "corrective emotional experience," that is, ". . . that the 'corrective'—or 'reconstructive'—value of the therapeutic experience is enhanced if the analyst's spontaneous reactions, the specific nature of his countertransference attitudes, or his studied attitudes are quite different from the original parental responses" (Alexander, 1961, p. 329-31). Alexander may not have intended to advocate deliberate role-playing by the analyst, but that is suggested by his phrase "studied attitudes." I do not believe that it is particularly helpful to patients to learn that other people can react differently than their parents did. Most patients have learned this already before coming into analysis. Even the intensification and enhancement of the experience of the analyst's differentness, for example, in the transference, is of doubtful therapeutic value. On the contrary, the analysand's experiencing the analyst as, at times, just as unempathic, or inappropriate, that is, just as deficient in providing needed selfobject responses as the parental selfobject was during early development, often leads to the kind of transference disruptions that allow a real working-through process to occur (Wolf, 1984a, 1985).[2]

But, as usual in psychoanalysis, matters are not quite that simple. Although specific studied attitudes and approbationary activities on part of the analyst are neither analytic nor therapeutic, it is paradoxically true that the analyst's own controlled regression in the analytic situation revives his own need for idealizable selfobjects, a need that leads to some overestimation of his analysand. The analysand will "experience this idealizing countertransference as a confirmation of his or her unrealized potential and as a stimulus to live up to it" (Wolf, 1983, p. 320).

2. Cf. Chapter 12.

.11.

COUNTERTRANSFERENCE ISSUES

THE ANALYSAND'S FEARS

Every self's ubiquitous need for self-sustaining selfobject responses would turn all of our social relations into moments of intimacy were it not for the equally omnipresent fears of self-fragmenting responses that force us to be always on the defensive. In the analytic situation, the demand of the basic rule to say everything that is thought, felt, and perceived—that is, to express verbally the totality of what is being experienced—is equivalent to a demand to suspend in thought and speech, though not in other behaviors, those rules that make a tolerable social life possible. It is, of course, an intolerable demand, and after long analytic work, the analysand's ability finally to comply signals that the analytic work has been largely accomplished. The protean forms in which resistance to complying with the basic rule manifests—they are among the most important resistances to analysis—paradoxically become the very substance that fuels the analytic process and thereby makes analysis possible. Particularly, transference, when defined as the patient's experience of the relationship (Gill & Hoffman, 1982), is linked to a fear-motivated resistance to complying with the basic rule. Yet without transference, psychoanalysis would be reduced to an empty shell of intellectualizations. There is little disagreement, therefore, among analysts about the central importance of analyzing the resistance we call transference, even though we may disagree about the priorities of timing (Gill & Hoffman, 1982; Wolf, 1984b). The term "resistance" may be misleading, because of its classical meaning in psychoanalysis, where it points to resistance against awareness of instinctual demands that are not acceptable to the superego. Within the theoretical context of self psychology, my use of the term "resistance" always means an activity motivated by fear of injury to the self and designed to protect the self's structure and boundaries.

THE ANALYST'S FEARS

Most analysts recognize that the analyst's self is similarly fearful of narcissistic injury and that the resulting defensiveness of the analyst could become a resistance to properly exercising the analyzing function. There is less agreement that the analyst is more than a mere observer and interpreting commentator, but an active participant in the analytic dialogue. His or her thoughts, feelings, and actions have an influence on the analytic process and on the patient that can usually be controlled but not altogether avoided. The analyst as a neutral blank screen is neither desirable nor attainable in the real world. The analyst's fear of injury to his or her self thus can become a hindrance to the analyst's functioning, that is, an undesirable countertransference.

Countertransference is just as ubiquitous as transference, sometimes as an obstacle, sometimes as a facilitator of the analytic process. Let us remember that the analyst is in a situation very similar to that of the analysand: There are constraints on the analyst's self-expression and a similar injunction to dismiss customary ways of thinking in favor of evenly hovering attention. These limitations and constraints combine to foster a regression in the analyst, which is not as intense as that of the analysand, and which is controlled, but which also mobilizes the analyst's selfobject needs. For example, an increased need for empathic "in tuneness" helps the analyst understand his or her patients better.

Gill (1982) states that the term "transference" and the phrase "the patient's experience of the relationship" are used interchangeably. I will adhere to the same usage and extend it also to the analyst's countertransference, where it will mean the *analyst*'s experience of the relationship. Thus described, transference and countertransference become equally important aspects of the analytic process, and we are encouraged to look at the analyst's participation in the analytic endeavor with his analysand without implying pathology. The concepts of transference and countertransference are means for approaching descriptively the subjectivities of both participants in the analytic situation. This allows us to talk about the dialectics of the analytic process or, in the words used by Atwood & Stolorow (1984, p. 119), about a system of interacting subjective worlds, which they term "intersubjectivity." I wonder whether one might not talk more clearly about a *dialectic of subjectivities*, leaning on Hegel's use of the term "dialectic" as the process by which contradictions are seen to merge themselves in a higher truth that comprehends them.

"Dialectic" seems a peculiarly apt term for talking about self–selfobject relations during analysis, where we can experience the contradictions between the subjectivities of self and selfobject merging themselves into an expanded and sometimes more highly organized self. No analyst can be totally neutral and free of bias with regard to his analysand. Even the well-analyzed analyst carries with him or her unanalyzed remnants of archaic expectations to be mirrored and to have idealizing selfobject responses available to him or her. Moreover, the exigencies of his or her daily existence press on the analyst and shape other conscious and unconscious expectations he or she will have *vis-à-vis* the analysand. In all of this the analyst is no different than the analysand, except, one may hope, that his self is stronger and more self-aware, which allows him to use himself more effectively and with less fear of losing his self. Rarely, specific weaknesses in the analyst's self may make him unsuitable as an analyst for a particular patient. Thus, as an example, an analyst's own needs to be mirrored, that is, his or her need for confirmatory selfobject responses, may have an undue influence on his intra-analytic behavior and interfere with the proper conduct of the analysis (Wolf, 1983, 1984b).

The Analyst's Vulnerabilities

An analyst's excessive need for mirroring may be rooted in (1) a persistent and excessive archaic remnant of selfobject needs distorted by a faulty selfobject milieu during early development, or (2) an enhancement of normally and usually expectable needs for mirroring because excessive frustration in the analytic situation has led to the analyst's regressing beyond what is desirable for a creative use of empathy. The latter frustration may result from: (a) The patient may be self-absorbed in his or her own needs for mirroring to the exclusion of any attention to the analyst's need to be addressed as a person as well. Such a patient deals with the analyst merely as another piece of "furniture" in the room that is at the patient's disposal. (b) The analyst may be defending against a patient's idealization of him or her, a defensiveness that makes the analyst assume a distant, cool, and aloof posture, which deprives him or her of the needed mirroring closeness to the patient. (c) The analyst may need to function competently the way he or she was taught an analyst should function when, as happens so often, a certain patient's fears and defensiveness seem to become obstacles to the smooth unrolling of the analytic process, leaving the analyst to doubt his or her own competence and appearing to threaten him or her with loss of professional standing. (d) Finally, the analyst's extra-analytic life may be so traumatically frustrating that the overburdened self of the analyst may be unable to satisfactorily fulfill its analytic functions.

None of these possibilities just enumerated ought to be thought of as pathology, but as recognizable contingencies that the analyst can work through to his or her own benefit as well as increasing his or her insight into and mastery of the dialectic of the analytic process in which analyst and analysand are involved. The analytic process involves both participants—they both get analyzed, so to speak. On infrequent occasions the countertransference cannot be worked through, and continues to disrupt the analytic process without restoration of the working relationship via interpretation. If the analyst's self-analysis of his or her self's malfunctioning produces no significant correction, then referral to another analyst may be indicated.

CLASSIFICATION

The classification of transferences and countertransferences presents a problem, because different theorists have approached this topic from different stances. Many analysts, therefore, lump together the totality of the intra-analytic experiences of the two participants respectively as "transference" or "countertransference."[1]

However, confusion may result when we lump together the transferences and countertransferences proper—that is, transferred

---

1. Gill and Hoffman (1982, p. 4) apparently solve this dilemma as far as "transference" is concerned by stating, "The term 'transference' and the phrase 'the patient's experience of the relationship' are used interchangeably throughout . . ." Gill and Hoffman stress that all "conflictual and resisted" aspects of the patient's experience are safely regarded as transference. They categorically reject any attempt to distinguish transference and nontransference on the grounds that the former "has either no basis or only a trivial basis in current reality, whereas the latter is reality-based."

from the past—with the reactions that are primarily evoked by the here-and-now situation.

Vignette A: A patient told her therapist about advising a friend to be hospitalized. She also mentioned her loneliness now, and the therapist interpreted her anxiety about losing the selfobject responsiveness that her friend had provided for her. In the subsequent session, the patient reported some regressive actions and seemed rather cold and annoyed. Associations led to the recognition that the patient had felt slighted by the therapist's interpretations of separation anxiety regarding the selfobject functions of the now hospitalized friend. Rather, she was angry because the therapist had not credited her skill and persuasive powers, which had been instrumental in getting her friend, in the face of great reluctance, into the hospital. An added slight was the fact that the therapist had suggested some days before that her friend might be better off hospitalized and now had not acknowledged the patient's exemplary behavior.

In this vignette one can discern the contributions of the patient's past—her need for continuous affirmation and recognition, a variety of mirror transference—and the therapist's contribution, in that his empathy failed to be attuned to the patient's need for a mirroring response. This is not to say that he should have praised her for her behavior, but he should have acknowledged her need for such affirmation, which at the time was greater than her need for staying close to her friend. The therapist also might have linked the patient's need for acknowledgment to certain childhood events and meanings that were known to both of them.

The contribution of the transference proper—that is, the archaic need for confirming selfobject experiences—and the contribution of the reaction to the therapist's faulty "in tuneness"—that is, the misleadingly termed "empathic failure"—can both be discerned. In my judgment, the archaic component contributed by the patient is an important aspect of her personality, and one must expect that, sooner or later, it will be drawn into the therapeutic process with the patient's becoming aware of its meaning. In contrast, even though it was the decisive trigger for the whole interactive experience, the therapist's "empathic failure" was probably rather expectable. On balance, therefore, I would judge this to have been a manifestation primarily of a proper transference rather than a reaction to the therapist.

Its analysis, however, would be contingent on first acknowledging the therapist's contribution—that is, his not having been attuned to the patient's meaning and thus having played a part in the precipitation of the disruptive events. Only then, after experiencing herself as an accepted participant, would the patient be able to also become enough of an observer of her own thoughts, feelings, and actions in both their contemporary form as well as in their archaic contexts, to gain therapeutic benefit from the disruptive experience. The increment of "cure" would not be the result of verbal interpretations or explanations, but a result of re-experiencing archaic traumatic constellations with a stronger, more resourceful self. The latter would find its strength in the selfobject experience made possible by the appropriate analytic ambience fortified by the attitude of reason as expressed in attempts to explain and interpret.

Vignette B: A patient who had been in treatment for a number of years mentioned during a session that her daughter, who lives out-of-town, was visiting and would be in the waiting room. The patient at that time was in an intense idealizing transference, proud of being associated with her therapist and proud of her successful daughter. After the session, the therapist just briefly nodded hello to the young woman whom he presumed to be the patient's daughter; then he returned to his office without giving the patient much of a chance to introduce him to the daughter. The following session with the patient was characterized by the patient's disappointment in the therapist, which she experienced as depression and anger for his not having let himself meet her daughter.

In this vignette, the contributions of both patient and therapist can also be observed. The patient's self needed the selfobject experience of being associated with an idealized selfobject. The therapist's avoidance of the patient's daughter was experienced by the patient as neither her self nor her daughter being deemed worthy of interest by the therapist. Ordinary expectable social courtesy would have demanded that the therapist allow the patient to introduce him to the daughter and to exchange some routine friendly greetings. His refusal to do so would have been thought rude in any other situation and, indeed, was rude in this situation as well.

Though the therapist rationalized his behavior as proper neutrality and abstinence, there were also other, more personal fears involved in the determination of his behavior. In this case, he was avoiding becoming annoyed if the next patient, who also was in the waiting room, should question him about this social interaction. Instead of analyzing whatever reaction the next patient might have, the analyst feared his own narcissistic vulnerability if he were criticized by that patient.

The patient's expectation to introduce him was also overdetermined by both ordinary courtesy as well as by her needs for idealizing selfobject experiences. The disappointment of the latter account for her depressive response, whereas the annoyance, a suppressed anger, was an appropriate reaction to the therapist's rudeness. The therapist, once he recognized his faulty attunement, should have acknowledged this to the patient without, however, sharing his insights into himself with the patient. Whether it would have been appropriate at that time to also interpret the patient's idealizing transference and her fear of expressing her anger is a matter of judgment as to timeliness and tact. Probably, it would be optimally productive to postpone the interpretation of the patient's part in this disruption to another, later session when the patient's self had recovered from the trauma of the experience. From the point of view of classification, this particular interaction would seem to consist of primarily a reaction to the therapist rather than a proper transference derived from archaic selfobject needs.

The Ubiquity of Transference and Countertransference

The constraints imposed on the patient by the therapeutic situation—that is, injunctions to refrain from ordinary social intercourse and action and instead to verbalize everything—is so different from the painfully learned modes of ordinary social life that these constraints cause a regression in the patient.

Analogous factors are also operative in the therapist, who similarly will experience some regressive pull. The therapist therefore will also experience some mobilization of repressed or disavowed strivings for self-fulfilment, with an intensification of his or her needs for certain selfobject experiences. Thus, the mobilization of countertransferences directed toward the patient is just as inevitable as the mobilization of the patient's transferences. The ubiquity of countertransferences is no more to be regretted than the analogous ubiquitous transferences. They both are equally essential aspects of the therapeutic process.

Nonspecific countertransferences are those expressions of more or less unconscious reactions of the therapist to the analytic situation and to being drawn into the analytic process as a participant. Prominent among these are the analyst's need to maintain control over his or her own self-structure to avoid too rapid or too severe regression.

Pleasure in Effectiveness

Any person's self-esteem is boosted by the pleasure one takes in one's own effectiveness. Indeed, even in very young infants it is easy to observe the spontaneous pleasure that erupts when the youngster succeeds in doing something he wants, for example, the joyful cries when seeing some specially sparkling toy or when manipulating some noisy bangle. These pleasures appear to be the rudimentary form of what in adults certainly are self-enhancing selfobject experiences: We all know the sense of self-satisfaction accompanied by a feeling of goodness and wholeness that we experience when we have succeeded in some difficult bodily or mental task. The strengthening of the self resulting from the selfobject experience of the exercise of our bodily or mental skills is probably related to the selfobject needs of the developing youngster. Whereas in the adult we can often analytically observe how the skillful accomplishment relates to an unconscious fantasy of being worthy of some idealized other or of being like an acceptable alter-ego—and, therefore, being acceptable oneself—it would be stretching the "adulto-morphizing" imagination to ascribe such fantasies to infants. Still, infants do seem to get strength from such experiences—and so do psychoanalysts from the properly successful exercise of their analytic skills.[2] (See also pages 60–62.)

2. Kohut has discussed the unhealthy effects of specialists' reliance upon and belief in the efficacy and accuracy of the tools/instruments and techniques of their discipline; such devotion to idealized methodologies isolates branches of science from each other and leads to rigidification internally with loss of vitality and of exploratory élan.

Countertransferences Proper

Countertransferences proper manifested by the therapist are mainly based on the analyst's residual archaic selfobject needs. By this I do not mean the normally expectable life-long needs for a modicum of mirroring, idealizing, and other selfobject experiences. I am referring, rather, to idiosyncratic needs that become mobilized in the treatment situation with certain particular patients. In these instances we do not only find the usual need for some recognition by the patient and the usual need to have a patient who is at least potentially admirable—in other words, the usual needs for some mirroring and for some idealizing—but we can observe quasi-pathological selfobject needs. For example, some patients can evoke the "scientist" in some therapists, who now must know everything, becoming a relentless seeker after the "truth" right now regardless of the cost in pain and discomfort. Such a therapist is not unlike the therapist who needs to be always right. A kind of fanatical dogmatism may pervade the therapeutic ambience as a sign that not all is well with the therapist. Insight into these countertransferences is usually all that is required to keep them under control, but when self-awareness or self-analysis are insufficient as a remedy, than some more formal analytic work may be the best solution.

Reactive Countertransferences

Countertransferences evoked by the patient's demands for selfobject experiences are another subcategory of the countertransferences. Some therapists find their patient's insistent demands for a mirroring selfobject experience intolerable, usually because it makes them feel impotent. Some therapists experience their patient's idealization of them as excessively stimulating to their own grandiose fantasies and either bear up with the discomfort or attempt to relieve their internal tension by some self-deprecatory comment. Many patients will feel painfully deprived of their need to have a selfobject experience with an idealized other, and such self-deprecation on the part of the therapist is both antitherapeutic and anti-analytic. A proper response is to analyze the patient's selfobject need with the patient, while simultaneously (and privately) analyzing one's own grandiosity and defensive denial. Some patients have the need to experience themselves as merged with the selfobject, a need that is an especially disconcerting selfobject transference for some therapists. These patients assume that the therapist knows what is on their mind, and that he shares their affective experience, their opinions, and judgments to the extent that the therapist feels he or she is no longer addressed as a separate person but has become a mere extension of the patient. For a therapist whose self is not too solidly cohesive, this experience may become threatening, and he or she will institute emergency protections for the self. The dogmatism and rigidity mentioned earlier are common defensive strategies.

. 12 .

ANALYTIC REALITY

OSTENSIVE AND DESCRIPTIVE KNOWLEDGE

The concept of an ostensive insight, which was introduced into psychoanalysis by the philosopher Jerome Richfield over 30 years ago, is seldom referred to in discussions of psychoanalytic reality. Richfield (1954) pointed out that we need to differentiate knowledge by acquaintance from knowledge by description. *Knowledge by acquaintance* is knowledge obtained without logical dependence on any inferential process or other knowledge of facts. For example, I have knowledge of both morphine and alcohol. I know that one is a bitter, white crystalline narcotic base; the other, I know to be a colorless, volatile, inflammable liquid that is intoxicating. But I know alcohol by acquaintance; morphine I know by description. That is, I have actually experienced the effects of alcohol: I have knowledge by direct acquaintance. This is specific knowledge, which no amount of discourse on the effects of alcohol could produce. I have no such direct cognitive experience of the effects of morphine, and what I know about it is only by analogy and inference. Richfield used the term *ostensive* to designate knowledge acquired by direct acquaintance with events that have occurred to a person.

Mutative Insights and Descriptive Insights

Richfield's distinction between ostensive and descriptive knowledge is of great importance in psychoanalysis because it helps us to clarify some crucial clinical issues. For by definition psychoanalysis deals with the data of inner experience that we call psychic reality, and our access to these data via introspection and empathy clearly marks our knowledge of psychic reality as an ostensive process, that is, as a process of knowing data by direct acquaintance. To be sure, when we are theorizing we can describe and talk about psychic reality as if it were something out there in the world. But the clinical meaning of the data of psychoanalysis can only be grasped ostensively, by direct experience.

In fact, that is what we mean by saying that introspection and empathy define and delimit the field of psychoanalysis. Therefore, I would suggest that the new analytic reality, which is constructed during a psychoanalysis by an analysand with the help of the analyst, will be different from the version of reality which the analysand brought into the analysis only to the extent that it was constructed out of ostensive knowledge acquired during analysis. Descriptive knowledge provided by the analyst will be effective only if it leads the analysand to experience something new—in other words, if it leads to direct acquaintance with subjectivities that become part of the process of constructing the new version of reality. Mutative insights—a concept introduced many years ago by James Strachey (1934)—consequently must be not merely descriptive insights, but ostensive insights. This means, for example, that interpretations made by the analyst will have little mutative power for the analysand unless they lead to an ostensive experience that is new and usually surprising to the analysand, and perhaps also to the analyst. Interpretations concerning a person who is emotionally very important carry a much greater likelihood of evoking a direct experience if the person happens to be present in the room at the time and is himself making the interpretation than if the interpretation concerns somebody far away in time and space, such as a deceased and well-mourned relative.

Superiority of Transference Interpretations

Considerations of this kind give some support to the contentions of those, like Gill (1982), who stress the primacy of transference interpretations over extratransference interpretations. However, it would be a mistake to conclude that transference interpretations are always superior to extratransference interpretations. The decisive question is not whether the interpretation is intra-analytic or extra-analytic, or about the transference or displaced from the transference; the decisive question is whether an interpretation leads to new knowledge by direct acquaintance that is, is experienced as ostensives, rather than being descriptively about something. Thus in many analyses, and often for a long time, defenses against the transference and defenses against being aware of the transference make transference interpretations quite useless, because they are experienced as descriptive and not ostensive. Early in the analysis, therefore, extratransference interpretations concerning immediate and highly charged extra-analytic relationships are likely to be experienced as more ostensively direct; therefore, they are likely to be more effective until resistance to awareness of the transference has diminished enough to make transference interpretations optimally profitable. One could define the task of the analyst in the analytic situation as bringing about new ostensive knowledge through the skillful use of interpretations.

Mutative Interpretations and Corrective Emotional Experience

Though this sounds at first very much like the time-honored prescription of insight through interpretation, I think I have made it clear that mere information is not enough; the evocation of a lived experience is required. I am not, however, as I have already noted, advocating a return to Alexander's "corrective emotional experience." The experience of an ostensive truth in a present relationship is something totally different from experiencing a role played by the analyst, as advocated by Alexander. Alexander hoped that patients would experience him as different from the way they had experienced their parents in childhood, and toward this end Alexander would purposefully try to be different than he understood a patient's parents to have been. Alexander attempted to play an emotional role that would be different from the emotional role of the parent and thereby provide a corrective emotional experience. In contrast, the ostensively direct experiences that I am suggesting as a necessary part of mutative interpretations are effective not because the analyst is so different from the parent, but because these ostensive experiences lead to new constructions of reality in spite of the fact that the analyst is experienced momentarily as being just as frustrating and distant and nonunderstanding as the parent was.

Such new reality constructions are indeed most useful, because the ostensive experience with the analyst was so very much like the archaic experience with the parent, but the self of the analysand is stronger now than in childhood and more capable of constructing a new reality in harmony with his own self structure, instead of being forced to accept the parent's reality as his own. The analyst is different from the parent of childhood in his or her empathic understanding of the analysand's legitimate and inevitable need to experience the analyst's minor and even trivial empathic failures as excruciating and often humiliating traumas.

Thus, the major significant difference between the traumatic archaic experience with the caregivers of early childhood and the therapeutic quality of the here-and-now experience with the analyst is the latter's acceptance of the analysand and of his or her experience as a legitimate experience among many possible legitimate experiences. To accept the analysand's experience as legitimate does not require that the analyst have the same experience. Nor does it require of the analyst that he or she approve or agree with the analysand in his or her thoughts, fantasies, wishes, or plans. All that it requires of the analyst is that he or she recognize, understand, and accept the patient's experience of reality as a given without having to accept the patient's reality as his or her own reality. On the contrary, as I discuss shortly, the discrepancy between the analyst's and the analysand's experiences are the proper material for the interpretive work that accepts and explains both experiences as legitimately occurring. The calamity of childhood trauma that rejects the child's experience as "bad" results in the substitution of what Winnicott called a "false self" for the child's own "true self."

To summarize, the analyst's reality is often experienced by the analysand as just as strange and frightening as the child experienced the parent's reality. In childhood, however, these different experiences of what is real could not be accepted or even negotiated—neither by the child nor the parent—but somebody's view had to prevail. Usually that meant the parent's experience of reality was right and the child was wrong, with traumatic consequences. In the analytic situation, optimally, no such overtones of moral right and wrong exist, and any number of realities can be constructed, co-exist and be accepted by both.

DISCREPANCIES IN EXPERIENCE OF REALITY

How do new psychic realities come into being in psychoanalysis? I believe the most frequent and the most effective opening for constructing a new analytic reality occurs when a discrepancy exists between the analyst's and the analysand's respective experiences of the analytic situation. Inevitably, analyst and analysand interact with each other. And inevitably, they experience this interaction differently. Much as the analyst might attempt to understand correctly the patient's experience of an intervention—let us say an interpretation—the analyst, even the most unbiased analyst informed by empathy and guided by the most appropriate theory, will inevitably, sooner or later, misunderstand the patient's experience and misconceive the patient's mental processes. Clearly, one may guess at or infer another's version of reality, but one cannot know it. Analogously, the patient will inevitably misunderstand the analyst, misjudge the analyst's experience of the patient, misconstrue the analyst's intentions, and misread the analyst's real misunderstandings into an exaggerated half-truth/half-fiction to fit the patient's previously learned experience. Misunderstanding is inevitable, because two people perceive the same situation with differing points of view, from different vantage points, with different affective reactions, and therefore have a different experience of what is going on. It is not a question of who is right and who is wrong. Both are. It is the discrepancy in subjectivities that matters and must be analyzed, that is, must be understood by both. One may hope, perhaps, that the analyst's experience is less determined "by a concealed repetition of earlier experiences and relationships" (Sandler, 1976, p. 39)—after all, he or she has been analyzed—and more by the mutual goals of the here-and-now situation than that of the analysand. But there is little room for either participant in the analytic situation to claim superiority for his or her experience over that of the other. Because the purpose of the analysis is to analyze the analysand, one has to start with analyzing the patient's experience of the analyst and of the analytic situation, that is, the analytic ambience as experienced by the analysand. Therefore, in clinical practice, it becomes incumbent upon the analyst to first accept and confirm the patient's experience as legitimately occurring before proceeding to understand it and to subject it (and the patient) to a dissecting kind of scrutiny.

To start with questioning another's experience per se, for example, to suggest he is "really feeling or thinking something else," is to question another's sanity or honesty. When this is done, albeit inadvertently and with the best of intentions, by the authority represented by the analyst, the effect on the analysand and the analysis is often devastating. Such obvious technical errors occur more often than we usually care to admit and can be largely prevented by incorporating in our clinical theories the fact that our conceptualizations describe the relationship between two distinctly different experiences, that is, two distinctly different versions of reality.

Analyst's Participation

Most discussions of psychoanalytic treatment focus attention only on what is going on within the patient, that is, on the patient's psychodynamics. References to the "actual situation" acknowledge that the patient has perceptions that do not represent a transference of genetic material, that is, are not necessarily caused by the archaic psychodynamics of early childhood, although transferences may, of course, influence the way the present actuality is experienced. Although it is certainly correct to talk about the "actual situation" and to discuss the interaction between patient and analyst as resulting in a new experience for the patient, many discussions of the analytic process do not mention that the analyst is also experiencing something, indeed, something that is markedly different from the patient's experience. This discrepancy between the analyst's and the analysand's experiences can easily become a major stumbling block around which the analysis may be derailed. Our tradition of logical positivism makes us hesitate to leave the safe ground of being the objective observer of interactions and interrelationships. We fear we would contaminate the purity of our scientific observations by personal bias and by the unconscious projection of our unresolved conflicts if we allowed ourselves to become involved as participants rather than just commenting observers.

We know, of course, that we *are* active participants in the analytic relationship, whether we like it or not, and we might even admit, if pressed to it, that we participate in accord with our personality, and that our experience of this participation is affective as well as cognitive. But in much analytic writing one gets no real whiff or taste of this affective participation, no allusions to our participating subjectivity, but only the image of the objectively observing scientist. Beyond the formal acknowledgment of their importance, we usually hear little about the nature of the experiences of either analyst or analysand. Thus, what is experienced by both participants in this uniquely evocative analytic situation, determining to a large extent the course of the analytic endeavor, remains a peripheral issue rather than becoming the center of our attention in elucidating transference and countertransference possibilities. The intersubjective aspects of the interactions have not yet become scientifically respectable data, and one often hears these aspects of the work of an analyst referred to as the "art of doing analysis" for which tact is required.

In a different context I have described some of the common interactive reactions of analyst and analysand to each other (Wolf, 1979):

> . . . it seems clear that the selfobject transferences consist of more than the reactivation of archaic forms of the persisting needs for selfobjects. Amalgamated with the reactivated archaic needs are the expectable age-appropriate selfobject needs of the analysand . . . that may easily be mistaken for resistances. Second, the analytic situation facilitates regression, and, as a result, the more archaic forms of needs for selfobjects become very prominent. . . . Third, analysts often become aware introspectively of an equally nonspecific reaction to the patient's initial reluctance. The analyst's reaction is derived from his healthy narcissistic involvement in his analytic work and from a misperception of the analysand as "resisting the analysis". . . . The analyst, just like the analysand, enters the analytic situation with certain needs for selfobjects. To be sure, it is expected that the analyst's own analysis has allowed him to work through the more archaic forms of his needs. . . . Still, after all is said and done, there always remain unfulfilled longings to be mirrored and unfulfilled strivings to merge. . . . Selfobject countertransferences, therefore, are an indispensable part of psychoanalytic treatment since they provide the major channel for those empathically collected data which make the formulation of psychoanalytic hypotheses possible. (pp. 585–86)

Atwood and Stolorow (1984, p. 41) have summarized

> . . . that psychoanalytic treatment seeks to illuminate phenomena that emerge within a specific psychological field constituted by the intersection of two subjectivities—that of the patient and that of the analyst.

In this conceptualization, psychoanalysis is not seen as a science of the intrapsychic, focused on events presumed to occur within one isolated "mental apparatus." Nor is it conceived as a science of the interpersonal, investigating the "behavioral facts" of the therapeutic interaction as seen from a point of observation outside the field under study. Rather, psychoanalysis is pictured here as a science of the *intersubjective*, focused on the interplay between the differently organized subjective worlds of the observer and the observed. The observational stance is always within, rather than outside, the intersubjective field or "contextual unit" (Schwaber, 1979) being observed, a fact that guarantees the centrality of introspection and empathy as the method of observation. (p. 41)

Whose Reality?

In a properly conducted analysis, it seems to me, the discrepancies in subjective experience between analyst and analysand are bound to become the foci of the working-through process. An examination of the discrepancies will reveal how much the influence of the past has contributed to the particular interpretation of the present relationship between analyst and analysand. Not only the analysand's subjective experience of the here-and-now is colored by the past in such a way as to give the present an often idiosyncratically shaded meaning for him; the same also is true of the analyst's subjectivity and, thus, for the interpretations he feels moved to make. Therefore, therapists are well advised to avoid interventions that imply either participant is distorting or is having inappropriate or incorrect experiences, because they are inappropriate only from the other's point of view.

In this way the analyst creates an analytic ambience in which the discrepancies of differing subjectivities can become discernible, understandable, and explainable—in other words, analyzable. Ideally, by focusing on the discrepancies, the investigation will begin to involve the analysand as a partner, not necessarily equally skilled in the mutual analytic endeavor, but equally respected for his or her essential contributions to the analytic process. Understanding the discrepancies between the two versions of reality as inevitable differences in meaning derived from their different experiences allows both participants to accept each other's interpretations, not unconditionally, but as appropriate within their individually different contexts.

The analyst's empathic perceptions of the patient's experience will then eventually be matched by the patient's increasing empathy for the analytic task performed by the analyst. The newly constructed analytic reality will then have three components: (1) the analysand's reality, mainly private but to some extent accessible to the analyst by empathy; (2) the analyst's reality, mainly private, but to some extent accessible to the analysand by empathy; and (3) the shared mutual reality of the understood and explained discrepancy between the two. This shared mutual reality, as it expands, guarantees an aspect of here-and-now actuality and thus acts as a preventive against either participant going off into the wild blue yonder of solipsism.

Appropriate mutual acceptance of all three constituents of analytic reality is equivalent to empathy at the highest level and strengthens the self cohesion of both parties. With their newly gained strength, the selfs of both may be able to accept even their own shortcomings and be willing to analyze them. By gaining the strength to really see what they have been looking at, both participants benefit from new perceptions that become part of the construction of a new reality for each—the analytic reality.

I would like now to report one case vignette to illustrate:

According to one particular patient, his history was remarkable, because each time some misfortune befell him the final outcome would always be to his advantage. He attributed this happy turn of events to "luck," and he carried the conviction that he was one of those people who were always blessed by a good luck that would rescue them from disasters.

I am tempted to label this view of reality a "myth of magic." It seems to represent a subvariety of Kris's (1956) "personal myth."

The list of happenings that were at first experienced with much distress but later seen by the patient to really have been instances of luck covered many areas of his life. But it was especially in the sphere of personal achievement that the "myth of magic" seemed to turn failure into success.

For example, the patient as a teenager and young adult had been fired from a number of jobs in which he had believed himself to be performing outstandingly well. Close analytic review of his performance on these jobs demonstrated that notwithstanding an adequate level of technical skill and competence, his arrogant know-it-all attitude had made him *persona non grata* to boss and coworkers. Immediately on getting fired he had become depressed, with some vague inkling that his grandiose self-overvaluation and the consequent poor interpersonal relationships he suffered were somehow connected to losing the job. Soon, however, a new job, perhaps with more pay or better hours or whatever, allowed him to again reconstruct this piece of life history as another instance of luck—in this case the good luck of having been fired leading to a better job. He had grown up in Eastern Europe, where he and his family had been engulfed by the disasters of war in which many relatives perished. Having managed to escape to the Western hemisphere he felt, of course, very lucky to have survived. But his personal conception of this lucky escape meant much more than mere survival. Indeed, as luck would have it, the disaster had propelled him into such fortunate circumstances in his adopted country that he now thought himself to be much better off than if the war had never occurred at all. This latter thought he admitted only with a great deal of shame about his having benefited from a series of events that had meant death and destruction to a large part of his family. A further symptom he reported was a slight feeling of unease whenever he was praised for some real achievement: He would insist on it being "just luck, nothing special, just being at the right place at the right time." Lady Luck protected him from shame and loss of self-esteem resulting from real as well as fancied failures.

The patient had grown up the eldest of four children, of which only a sister two years his junior played a distinct role in his early life. Her birth one day before his own second birthday remained a source of continuing aggrievedness throughout childhood, because the long-awaited celebrations of his sister's birthdays always seemed to overshadow his birthday party the next day and made him feel less important than her. He found a measure of consolation for this painful blow to his self-esteem in his ability to provoke her into tears of humiliation by his using his more mature intellectual and physical skills. He even managed these provocative actions in a way that escaped the notice of his mother, so that he avoided blame while the sister was chided for her babyish crying. At the same time, as the oldest and only boy, he clearly felt that he was mother's favorite and could manipulate her to take his side and protect him in all controversies. The relationship with his father was more openly ambivalent. Father's once thriving business had failed during the Great Depression when the patient was eight years old. The father was now reduced to accepting a less important position in the family business that had passed into the hands of his oldest brother.

Compared with his uncles on both sides of the family, the patient's father seemed kinder and more intelligent, but rather ineffectual. A further obstacle in the patient's need to idealize his father was the father's history of having been sickly as an adolescent and having terminated his education before graduation from highschool. In consequence of this family constellation, the patient entered upon adolescence with a deficient self structure: A too early and too severely abrupt disillusionment in his father had disrupted an appropriately evolving response to his archaic idealizing selfobjects needs and had left his self with an area of fragility at the pole of ideals and values. Characteristically, he was constantly searching for strong men, especially among teachers, to find a source for needed idealizing selfobject responsiveness. Although he was vaguely aware of always feeling somewhat inferior to his cousins and friends, he constructed a self-image of secret intellectual superiority. In this he was encouraged by his mother, who rarely ever criticized him for his social awkwardness, but voiced her strong conviction in a future successful professional career that she envisaged for him. When a growing sense of reality forced him to recognize the flaws in mother's idolization of him, he displaced the needed mirroring selfobject function onto his version of Lady Luck.

Illusory Versions of Reality

We can discern here a shift from a miscarried idealizing selfobject function—resulting from the disappointment in the father who failed him—to a compensatory and well-functioning mirroring selfobject function carried by his mother, and, later, symbolized by luck as a compensatory structure. From this, he constructed a particular but skewed version of reality. But although this compensatory structure magically helped him over many a rough spot, it also propelled him into self-defeating arrogance. We can say that he repeatedly ignored certain aspects of his relationship to his surround so that he could maintain the belief of being under the special protection he called luck. Kris's patient, like mine, created his own psychic reality by selecting from past experiences those which best fit into the self-image he needed to feel good about himself. Let us call this activity the creation of an illusory version of reality. Analysands (the others) experience such illusions as the absolute truth.

REALITY OR ILLUSION: A REEXAMINATION
OF KRIS'S CONCEPT OF THE "PERSONAL MYTH"

The preceding discussion highlights the vicissitudes and subjective nature of what a person may call "reality." To paraphrase an old proverb, it seems that one man's reality is another man's illusion. Ernst Kris (1956) made an important contribution to the discussion of these issues. It is appropriate to reexamine his concept of the "Personal Myth" here from the point of view of the special concerns of a clinical theory framed by psychoanalytic self psychology. Not only "reality" or "illusions" but even "memories" are created by the individual in response to individual psychological needs, as already apparent to Kris (1956, pp. 297-98):

> . . . the selective character of what traditionally is called the period of infantile amnesia. It includes the experiences of the self, but does not include the impact of reality testing, skills, conceptualization or information acquired during the same period of time. In all those areas where the self is concerned, where memory is autobiographical, autonomy in the broadest sense is never fully achieved, distorting influences never cease to play their part, and recollections remain connected with needs and affects. (pp. 297-98)

Screen Memories

Freud (1899) in his "Screen Memories" focused on what is remembered rather than on what is omitted and suggested, as Kris did in the "Personal Myth," the purpose for recasting memories:

> . . . close investigation shows rather that these falsifications of memory are tendentious—that is they serve the purposes of repression and replacement of objectionable or disagreeable impressions. (p. 322)

But one further comment by Freud (1899) assumes increasing significance as we re-examine the process of creating the autobiographical self-image out of memories:

> Above all, there is the following point. In the majority of significant and in other respects unimpeachable childhood scenes one sees one's own person in the recollection as a child, with the knowledge that this

child is oneself; one sees this child, however, as an observer from outside the scene would see him. . . . Now it is evident that such a picture cannot be a faithful repetition of the impression that was originally received. For at that time one found oneself in the middle of the situation and was attending not to oneself but to the external world. . . .

Whenever in a memory one's own person appears in this way as an object among other objects this contrast between the acting and recollecting self may be taken as evidence that the original impression has been worked over. (p. 321; my translation)

Psychic Reality and Objective Reality

Freud's last comment here implies that all autobiographical memories in which one's own person appears as an object among objects must have been worked over, and, therefore, are in some sense bound to be different than the original experience. This observation challenges the possibility of ever describing accurately as "an observer from outside the scene" what the remembered experience in question really was. It raises the important issue of psychic reality versus so-called objective reality. Freud saw clearly that even in our memories we usually repress the recollection of the psychic reality as it was experienced in favor of reconstructing in harmony not only with the purposes of repression to eliminate disagreeable impressions, but also in harmony with the so-called objective reality that the outside world and our reality testing imposes on us. Clearly, two realities vie for our attention and allegiance; neither can be designated as true or false by any criteria acceptable to everyone.

Choosing Reality

Because there seems to be no absolute true reality, but as many realities as there are observers observing from various locations in psychic space and time, we must choose and define our "reality." It is my thesis that the differences between "classical" psychoanalytic interpretations and self-psychologically informed ones are based on having made a different choice among the realities vying for our allegiance. Kris's interpretations reflect his attempt to discern as closely as possible an objective reality as seen by an outside observer.

A self-psychological interpretation reflects an attempt to discern as closely as possible the reality of the patient's experience. It is comparable to two observers looking at the same landscape from different locations and through different kinds of telescopes. Their different views cannot possibly be the same, but they might both be correct. Thus, we must choose our observing instrument, that is, our theory.

Usually, however, we do not recognize that we have made a choice, because our direct experience of our senses or our memory seems so strong and self-evident that we blithely call any other view that conflicts with our own choice as false. Freud (1899) chose the outside observer's reality as his criterion of truth:

> Out of a number of childhood memories of significant experiences, all of them of similar distinctness and clarity, there will be some scenes which, when they are tested (for instance by the recollections of adults), turn out to have been falsified. (p. 322)

Freud's Choice

Thus when Freud (1899) uses the word "falsification" (p. 322) or Kris uses the term "duplicity" (p. 276) in connection with his analysand, we can discern a commitment to the observer's truth and, in Kris's (1956) instance, even to the observer's morality. Freud (1914) stated his choice also quite clearly when discussing the attitude of affectionate parents toward their children. He noticed their

> . . . compulsion to ascribe every perfection to the child—which sober observation would find no occasion to do—and to conceal and forget all his shortcomings. . . . Illness, death, renunciation of enjoyment, restrictions on his own will, shall not touch him; the laws of nature shall be abrogated in his favor; he shall once more really be the centre and core of creation—"His Majesty the Baby," as we once fancied ourselves. (p. 91)

Subjective Experience at the Core

Freud thought, as every outside observer must think, that the parental attitude he described resulted from an overvaluation of the child quite in contrast to "sober observation." But he also acknowledges the baby's experience—"as we once fancied ourselves"—as being at the centre and core of creation.

Let us look briefly at the baby's experience of blissful omnipotence or at an adult patient's experience of omnipotent power. What attitude shall we take toward such assertions, whether they are verbally stated or enacted in the transference or just surmised empathically? Do we agree that their self-perceptions are correct? Or do we examine the evidence for their beliefs? Or do we try to find out the meaning of their perceptions and beliefs? Is it at all possible to take an attitude that does not lean on some view of reality that we hold as a criterion of truth?

Analyst's Choice

I believe we can and must choose to accept the analysand's perceptions and beliefs as true, even though we know they are shaped by his or her experiences, biases, and unreliable memory, as well as by all kinds of conscious and unconscious motivations. We must accept the analysand's truth, because only by accepting as true what he or she experiences as true can we begin the analytic dialogue that will determine the meaning of this truth—that is, will make it clear to analysand as well as to analyst that this truth is not absolute, but relative to the context in which it was experienced. Thus, a path is opened to an ever-widening sphere in which experiences can be seen and evaluated from many points of view.

The analyst's empathic stance *vis-à-vis* the analysand can become the latter's empathic stance *vis-à-vis* his or her whole life experience. At a suitable time it may perhaps be appropriate to educate the analysand to recognizing that others may experience a different truth, but almost invariably he or she knows that already and is likely to perceive such educational efforts as insulting his or her intelligence. Because the actuality of the past, how it happened and how it was experienced, is never ascertainable with any high degree of reliability, let us admit this state and look upon the assertions in the present as communications about the present state of the communicator's psyche. "His Majesty the Baby" is telling us something about the present state of the baby's self. The analysand who conveys to us his deep feelings of worthlessness is similarly telling us something about the state of his self; and the analysand who enacts with us his conviction of being Superman also is telling us something about the state of his self. It is not our job to judge the truth value of someone else's reality by our standards of truth, nor is it our job to modify our patient's view of reality in order to bring it into conformity with our view of reality. It is our job to use whatever information we can gather about the analysand's state to help him recognize that state of his self, its self-expressiveness and its self-defensiveness, to help him detect the factors that brought it about, and to help him see what he can do to alter and to strengthen it. Then we can safely assume that the strengthened self will have less need to alter its perceptions in order to safeguard its fragile integrity. Indeed, as the analytic process leads to a strengthened self, one often observes a gradual change in the analysand's perception of reality, including his autobiographical image, bringing it more into harmony with the reality seen by the outside observer.

Relevant Reality

In self psychology we attempt to choose as the analysand's truth the analysand's experience of it. I have to say "attempt" because another's experience is not directly accessible, but only dimly graspable by vicarious introspection, that is, by empathy. We know the impossibility of introspecting the self state without bias, and our conclusions about self and others seem to lack the rich detail and the clear evidential data that characterize the outside observer's truth. But lack of scientific proof does not mean falsehood. The pivotal question is not the degree of reliable reproducibility, but its relevance to the problem at hand. Our choice to pursue the elusive truth of subjective experience rather than that of objective observation is grounded in our belief in its more immediate relevance to the psychoanalytic enterprise. The great majority of our analyzable patients need not be educated to the reality around them nor to the manner in which they are being perceived by their surround. Instead, we try to revive and make conscious, albeit usually most imperfectly, the repressed and disavowed experiences of early life as those experiences modify perceptions of self and others and as they reveal themselves through being re-enacted in the here-and-now. To do this we must enter into the patient's reality, the reality that often appears to the outside observer as illusion.

Scientific Objectivity

We must approach the "personal myths" of our patients with a similar attitude of accepting the reality of their experience. In a previous publication, (Wolf, 1980-1981), I tried to show that as psychoanalysts we must attempt to grasp not only the hard truths of the objective scientist, but also the soft and more subjective truths of the artist. The latter truths are not as easily demonstrated to a skeptical and scientifically trained public, but that does not make them any less truthful. Above all, we must avoid the prejudice of our contemporary era that labels as false what the scientist cannot prove beyond doubt. We need the poetic faith of which Coleridge spoke as the willing suspension of disbelief for the moment. Scientific objectivity and poetic faith need not be antagonistic, but can be brought together into a synthesis—or dialectic, if you like—that can illuminate human life.

The ideal of objectivity, that is, the control of the unavoidable influence of the individual observer on the observed, is just as important in psychoanalysis as in physics. In physics, when dealing with the macrostructures of daily life, these influences can be ignored as insignificant because they are so very small. It is only when observing the microstructures of the smallest particles that the observer's effect becomes significant. How about psychoanalysis? Kohut (1977, p. 31n.) suggests that in this respect the transactions of the clinical situation are analogous to observation in the realm of the smallest particles in physics as far as the influence of the observer on the observed is concerned (pp. 36-38).

Absolute or Relative Truth

Freud (1933) saw things differently. For him, truth was something absolute, not relative:

> The ordinary man only knows one kind of truth, in the ordinary sense of the word. He cannot imagine what a higher or a highest truth may be. Truth seems to him no more capable of comparative degrees than death; and he cannot join in the leap from the beautiful to the true. Perhaps you will think as I do that he is right in this. (p. 172)

Grandiose Illusions

The analysand whom I reported as having created the mythical good luck in his autobiography reminds one of Freud's (1908b) reference to a fictional character in an early paper. Anzengruber's *Steinklopferhans* flouted all dangers with the parole "Nothing can happen to *me*."

> . . . through this revealing characteristic of invulnerability we can immediately recognize His Majesty the Self, the hero alike of every day-dream and of every story. (p. 150; my translation)

His Majesty the Self, which Freud later referred to as His Majesty the Baby (1914, p. 91), are typical of experienced realities that from an outside observer's point of view are illusions. Both views are correct from the vantage point of the respective experiencing observers. Difficulties arise when one attempts to impose one view of reality on the other. To question another's perceptions arouses anxiety at the least, and can be destructive at its worst.

Developmental Considerations

Kohut (1978, p. 438) quoted from Trollope's novel *Barchester Towers* a description of the rapturous relationship between mother and infant. Indeed, a mutual admiration of mother and infant regularly attends what is fairly called an experience of blissful well-being. Though the baby at this time cannot be credited with any thought content, the total experience is equivalent to an illusion of unique and superlative excellence, an illusion usually shared by the mother even though she may, on reflection, know better. His Majesty the Baby (Freud, 1914, p. 91) is an apt term for this grandiose illusion that is willingly entered into by both infant and parent, that is, by the self-selfobject unit, even if only for the brief moment that whispers, "Here we are, together, the most beautiful child and the most perfect parent." I believe such grandiose but illusory experiences are a necessary requirement for the normal and healthy development of self and self-esteem. An over dedication to reality on part of the parents will lead to premature debunking of the child's exaggerated beliefs about itself by pointing out, in the name of having to learn about the real world, the child's smallness, weakness, vulnerability, and other shortcomings. In this way the developing self is crushed and crippled, with future self disorder an ordained conclusion. The values of the scientific laboratory—the cold, hard facts—are superbly productive of scientific truths, but totally unsuited to allowing the creation of the human qualities of life.

Ubiquitous Illusions

Similar considerations must govern the analytic ambience if it is to facilitate the healing of an injured self. Freud's total commitment to an absolute truth as he saw it prevented him from fully harvesting all his rich insights into the creative and curative process. For he failed to appreciate fully that the infantile illusion was, indeed, for the child a reality that is absolutely necessary for the establishment of the child's firm sense of selfhood; and, analogously, as adults we harbor some illusions that are necessary for us to function effectively. The most common of these probably is the illusion of immortality. To be sure, we all "know" that someday we must die. But I have yet to meet the person to whom this knowledge about existence is a living and experienced reality—with the possible exception of some people who actually are close to death. No matter how much of the actuality of the real world outside of us we believe and accept and let regulate our behavior in that world, there still remains a psychic reality—equally true though illusory to others—in which we *live* and which we reject at the peril of our sanity. Freud (1908b) thought that the child distinguishes his world of play and fantasy quite well from reality:

> . . . the child at play . . . creates a world of fantasy which he takes very seriously—that is, which he invests with large amounts of emotion— while separating it sharply from reality. (p. 144)

Separation of Reality from Illusion

But I believe the separation is not quite as sharp as Freud thought. The tangible and visible things of the world have selfobject functions that make them part of our selves and thus restore to us, or sometimes even give us *de novo*, our wholeness. As the child becomes an adult, he believes more and more, in harmony with everyone else, that reality resides outside and that inside are fantasies, imagination—in short, illusions. He no longer knows and usually does not remember that in his innermost being, his nuclear self, he still lives in that inside reality.

It is doubtful to me that we can do justice to our analysands if we believe that their autobiographical self-images are merely in the service of hiding sexuality and aggression and that therefore we are dealing with falsifications and duplicities. The "personal myths" that our patients reveal to us must be treated with the respect and gentleness required by the fragile selfs of which they are an expression.

· 13 ·

TERMINATION

Many questions arise in connection with termination of a depth-psychological treatment. When is a patient ready for termination? How should termination be initiated? What are the characteristic phenomena of the termination process? (Cf. Shane & Shane, 1984.)

When analyst and analysand have been working together, more or less successfully, for a number of months that usually add up to a few years, the goal of a strengthened self will probably have been reached and the question of termination comes up. In this context termination means the cessation of the formal, four or five times per week regularly scheduled analytic sessions. However, in a certain sense the analytic process, if it was successful, will go on within the analysand—and, of course, also within the analyst—in the form that has been termed a selfanalytic process. Indeed, the continuing analysis of the self by the self, for the rest of one's lifetime, is one of the indications of a successful analytic experience. In this special sense, therefore, there is no termination of the analysis.

However, we are considering the termination of the formal analytic sessions of analyst and analysand. How do analyst and analysand decide when and how to terminate their formal analytic relationship? Usually it is the patient who first raises the question of termination. The patient may be motivated to initiate this discussion by a more or less appropriate desire to bring treatment to an end, or because he or she fears that the therapist may be contemplating termination, perhaps prematurely. Sometimes the therapist will begin discussion of possible termination because he or she has become convinced that the patient has obtained optimal benefit from the treatment but does not wish to leave the security of the relationship.

I think it is important to recognize that both patient and therapist always will experience a resistance to terminating if they have had a satisfactory and productive working relationship over a long period of time. Experienced therapists are likely to be aware of any unconscious tendencies to prolong treatment unnecessarily and will take corrective action. Both participants in a creative analytic dialogue derive selfobject experiences that strengthen the structure of their selfs. Yet, some anxieties, depressions and conflicts remain. They are part of life, no matter how well analyzed the person may be. But one hestitates to end a relationship that has been helpful to the analysand.

In my experience, it has been the emergence in the analysand of self-analytic skills combined with a mobilization of creative activities and increasing ease and satisfaction in social relationships that signal the approach of a timely termination. Kohut (1966) looked for creativity, empathy, a capacity to contemplate one's own impermanence, a sense of humor, and wisdom as the signs of a transformed narcissism. Transference and countertransference aspects need to be analyzed when they interfere with the proper initiation and progress of the termination process.

The question of when to terminate would be easier to answer if one could point to a set of generally agreed-upon criteria for termination. Therapists' criteria often seem to depend on the theory informing the treatment and are not necessarily in concert with the patient's goals. Analysands usually come into treatment with vaguely defined treatment goals, such as wanting to feel better, get along better with family or coworkers, be rid of certain behavioral or somatic symptoms, and the like. During the course of treatment some of these goals are reached, others may change, still others may turn out to be resistant to any substantial change but may become less important to the patient.

A lawyer in his late thirties came into analysis because of frequent attacks of angry shouting when frustrated by clients. These episodes of narcissistic rage endangered not only his job, but also his relationship with his wife, whom he might treat with cold contempt when she failed to live up to his unrealistic expectations. He felt ready to terminate after about four years of analysis when the rageful outbursts had disappeared completely and when the relationship with his wife had become much more mutually warm and supportive. During the analysis he had become aware of certain sensitivities related to vulnerable aspects of his self. Particularly, he had to recognize and accept that an archaic fear of being left and abandoned by significant persons in his selfobject surround was still present though much diminished and now rarely leading to symptoms. But the analytic experience had strengthened his self and left him with enough insights to be able to cope without the fragmentations that had previously endangered him. Termination was appropriate and timely. Still, it would have been possible to continue the analysis with the likely goal of even further reductions in anxiety–hostility.

The self-psychologically oriented therapist will pay close attention to the patient's therapeutic goals without necessarily adopting them as his own. If the patient wants to terminate prematurely— that is, before reaching reasonably attainable goals—because of fears emanating from the transference, the therapist must explain these fears and urge working through rather than acting out by terminating. Such explanations are not always successful:

A middle-aged psychiatrist came into treatment because his countertransference reactions to his patients were interfering with doing psychotherapy. Soon after treatment began he felt outraged when he was charged the same fee that other patients were charged. He felt that he was entitled to special consideration and was not satisfied by any of his therapist's explanations. He quit treatment before really getting started.

Most likely the therapist's countertransference also played a role in this miscarried attempt to start a workable treatment relationship. Perhaps the therapist's narcissism was wounded by this patient's presumption, and he might otherwise have been more effective in his explanations. Sometimes the combination of a particular patient's transferences with a particular therapist's countertransferences make a collaborative endeavor impossible. It is neither useful nor rational to try to place blame, but it is best to refer to another therapist.

Here is another example:

Toward the end of the first year of analysis, an analysand developed an intense erotic transference that caused her to feel restless and embarrassed because she felt herself unworthy of the attention that she longed for so much. When the therapist during this time announced his upcoming vacation, the patient missed the next appointment and phoned to cancel all other appointments, in effect terminating the treatment. The therapist persuaded her to come in for the next scheduled appointment and at that time explained to her that the intensity of her feelings, especially her feeling embarrassed by unacceptable desires, seemed to make it imperative to protect herself against the source of these emotions by distancing herself. In the ensuing weeks, enough working through could take place to avoid a premature termination.

As already stated, therapists' criteria for their patients' termination are influenced by the theoretical frame within which they are working. From the point of view of the psychology of the self, one may look for a strengthening of the self to the point where the self has become enabled to rely less on defensive maneuvers designed to protect the cohesion, boundaries, and vigor of the self. At the same time, aware of its increased resiliency and lessened vulnerability, the self has become more expressive of itself and more daring in its actions.

Six years after coming into treatment, a mother of three no longer feared that she would lose control over her rages and injure her children. She had discovered during her analysis how vulnerable she was to feeling slighted and threatened when she experienced her surround as not being interested in her. The experience of similar affects in the transference at times assumed almost traumatic intensity and were traceable to analogous traumatic experiences during childhood, precipitated in the analysis by some out-of-tune response from the analyst. Explanation of these disruptive experiences always restored the transference relation to a cooperative one, and the solidity gained allowed the patient to slightly restructure her life to avoid patently noxious relationships in favor of responsive ones. As a result, she became calmer, stronger, feeling less helpless and therefore less likely to experience narcissistic rage. She also had resumed an artistic creative hobby in which she found much satisfaction. Her need for soothing responsiveness, though diminished, remained, but, being less defensively distant from people, she was able to have the needed responsive experiences. The inevitable frustrations now found her calmer and stronger and better able to cope without losing control.

Once patient and therapist have agreed upon terminating their formal therapeutic relationship, they can decide on optimal timing. Almost always it is wise to set a termination date that allows several months of continuing working through, especially working through the very anxieties associated with termination itself. As the termination date comes closer, one can often notice some trepidation and a desire to postpone the feared day. Most of the time it is probably best to stick to the date that was set originally, but some flexibility permits one to correct errors in judgment regarding the original date for termination and also makes it possible to take into consideration new and possibly unforeseen circumstances.

Many patients feel the need for post-termination contact of some kind. Some will want to be able to phone for an occasional appointment, others just want to feel free to contact the therapist if they think it necessary. It is well to encourage staying in touch because it is in the spirit of an appropriately responsive relationship.

REFERENCES

Agosta, L. (1984). Empathy and intersubjectivity. In: *Empathy I*, ed. J. Lichtenberg, M. Bornstein, & D. Silver. Hillsdale, NJ: Analytic Press, 1984, pp. 43–61.

Alexander, F. (1958). Unexplored areas in psychoanalytic theory and treatment—Part II. In: *The Scope of Psychoanalysis*. New York: Basic Books, 1961, pp. 326–331.

——— (1961). *The Scope of Psychoanalysis*. New York: Basic Books.

Angyal, A. (1941). *Foundations for a Science of Personality*. New York: Commonwealth Fund.

Atwood, G., & Stolorow, R. (1984). *Structures of Subjectivity*. Hillsdale, NJ: The Analytic Press.

Bacal, H. (1985). Optimal responsiveness and the therapeutic process. *Progress in Self Psychology*, Vol. 1, ed. A. Goldberg. New York: Guilford Press, pp. 202–227.

Basch, M. F. (1983). Some theoretical and methodological implications of self psychology. In: *The Future of Psychoanalysis*, ed. A. Goldberg, New York: International Universities Press, pp. 431–442.

——— (1986). Can this be psychoanalysis? In: *Progress in Self Psychology*, Vol. 2., ed. A. Goldberg, New York: Guilford Press, pp. 18–30.

Beebe, B., & Lachmann, F. (1988). Mother–infant mutual influence and precursors of psychic structure. In: Frontiers in Self Psychology: *Progress in Self Psychology*, Vol. 3, ed. A. Goldberg. Hillsdale, NJ: Analytic Press, pp. 3–25.

Brandchaft, B. (1986). British object relations theory and self psychology. In: *Progress in Self Psychology*, Vol. 2., ed. A. Goldberg, New York: Guilford Press, pp. 245–272.

Broucek, F. (1979). Efficacy in infancy: A review of some experimental studies and their possible implications for clinical theory. *International Journal of Psychoanalysis*, 60:311–316.

Demos, E. V. (1988). Affect and the development of the self: A new frontier. In: *Frontiers in Self Psychology: Progress in Self Psychology*, Vol. 3, ed. A. Goldberg. Hillsdale, NJ: Analytic Press, pp. 27–53.

Ellenberger, H. F. (1970). *The Discovery of the Unconscious*. New York: Basic Books.

Fairbairn, W. R. D. (1944). Endopsychic structure considered in terms of object-relationships. In: *An Object-Relations Theory of Personality*. New York: Basic Books, 1952.

Fenichel, O. (1945). *The Psychoanalytic Theory of Neurosis*. New York: W. W. Norton.

Freud, S. (1895). Case histories. *Standard Edition*, 2:21–181.

171

—— (1899). Screen Memories. *Standard Edition*, 3:303-322.

—— (1900). The Interpretation of Dreams. *Standard Edition* 4 & 5.

—— (1905a). A Case of Hysteria. *Standard Edition*, 7:15-122.

—— (1905b). Three essays on the theory of sexuality. *Standard Edition*, 7:130-243.

—— (1908). Creative writers and daydreaming. *Standard Edition*, 9:142-153.

—— (1913a). Zur Einleitung der Behandlung. *Gesammelte Werke*, 8:454-478. Frankfurt a/M: S. Fischer, 1945.

—— (1913b). The disposition to obsessional neurosis. *Standard Edition*, 12:317-326.

—— (1914). On narcissism: An introduction. *Standard Edition*, 14:73-102.

—— (1920a). Beyond the pleasure principle. *Standard Edition*, 18:7-64.

—— (1920b). A note on the prehistory of the technique of analysis. *Standard Edition*, 18:263-265.

—— (1921). Group psychology and the analysis of the ego. *Standard Edition*, 18:69-143.

—— (1926). The question of lay analysis. *Standard Edition*, 20:183-250.

—— (1933). New introductory lectures on psychoanalysis. *Standard Edition*, 22:7-128.

Galatzer-Levy, R. (1988). Manic-depressive illness: Analytic experience and a hypothesis. In: *Frontiers in Self Psychology: Progress in Self Psychology*, Vol. 3, ed. A. Goldberg. Hillsdale, NJ: Analytic Press, pp. 103-142.

Gedo, M. (1980). *Picasso: Art as Autobiography*. Chicago: University of Chicago Press.

Gedo, J., & Pollock, G. (eds.) (1976). *Freud: The Fusion of Science and Humanism*. New York: International Universities Press.

Gill, M. (1982). *Analysis of Transference*. Vol. 1. New York: International Universities Press.

—— & Hoffman, I. (1982). *Analysis of Transference*. Vol. 2. New York: International Universities Press.

Goldberg, A. (ed.). (1978). *The Psychology of the Self: A Casebook*. New York: International Universities Press.

—— (ed.). (1980). *Advances in Self Psychology*. New York: International Universities Press.

—— (ed.). (1983). *The Future of Psychoanalysis*. New York: International Universities Press.

—— (1985). The definition and role of interpretation. In: *Progress in Self Psychology*, Vol. 1. New York: Guilford, pp. 62-65.

Grünbaum, A. (1984). *The Foundations of Psychoanalysis*. Berkeley: University of California Press.

Guntrip, H. (1961). *Personality Structure and Human Interaction*. New York: International Universities Press.

Hartmann, H. (1950). Comments on the Psychoanalytic theory of the ego. In: *Essays on Ego Psychology*. New York: International Universities Press, 1964, pp. 113-141.

Hendrick, I. (1942). Instinct and the ego during infancy. *Psychoanalytic Quarterly*, 11:33-58.

——— (1943). Work and the pleasure principle. *Psychoanalytic Quarterly*, 12:311–329.

Jones, E. (1954). *Hamlet and Oedipus*. New York: Doubleday.

Kohut, H. (1959). Introspection, Empathy and Psychoanalysis. In: *The Search for the Self*, ed. P. Ornstein. New York: International Universities Press, 1978, pp. 205–232.

——— (1966). Forms and transformations of narcissism. In: *The Search for the Self*, ed. P. Ornstein. New York: International Universities Press, 1978, pp. 427–460.

——— (1968). The Psychoanalytic Treatment of Narcissistic Personality Disorders. In: *The Search for the Self*, ed. P. Ornstein. New York: International Universities Press, 1978, pp. 477–509.

——— (1971). *The Analysis of the Self*. New York: International Universities Press.

——— (1972). Thoughts on Narcissism and Narcissistic Rage. In: *The Search for the Self*, ed. P. Ornstein. New York: International Universities Press, 1978, pp. 615–662.

——— (1976). Creativeness, Charisma, Group Psychology. In: *The Search for the Self*, ed. P. Ornstein. New York: International Universities Press, pp. 804–823.

——— (1977). *The Restoration of the Self*. New York: International Universities Press.

——— (1978). *The Search for the Self: Selected writings of Heinz Kohut: 1950–1978*, Vols. 1 & 2, ed. P. Ornsteinn. New York: International Universities Press.

——— (1982). Introspection, empathy and the semi-circle of mental health. *International Journal of Psychoanalysis*, 63:395–407.

——— (1984). *How Does Psychoanalysis Cure?* Chicago: University of Chicago Press.

——— (1985). *Self Psychology and the Humanities*. ed. C. Strozier. Chicago: University of Chicago Press.

——— & Wolf. E. S. (1978). The disorders of the self and their treatment. *International Journal of Psychoanalysis*, 59:414–425.

Kris, E. (1956). The personal myth. In: *The Selected Papers of Ernst Kris*. New Haven: Yale University Press, 1975, pp. 272–300.

Leider, R. (1983). Analytic neutrality. *Psychoanalytic Inquiry* 3:665–674.

Lichtenberg, J. (1983). *Psychoanalysis and Infant Research*. Hillsdale, NJ: Analytic Press.

——— (1989). *Psychoanalysis and Motivation* (in preparation).

Lichtenberg, J., & Kaplan, S. (eds.). (1983). *Reflections on Self Psychology*. Hillsdale, NJ: Analytic Press.

Meyers, S. (1988). On supervision with Heinz Kohut. In: *Frontiers of Self Psychology; Progress in Self Psychology*, Vol. 4, ed. A. Goldberg. Hillsdale, NJ: Analytic Press.

Miller, J. (1985). How Kohut actually worked. In: *Progress in Self Psychology*, Vol. 1, ed. A. Goldberg. New York: Guilford Press, pp. 13–30.

Miller, J., Sabshin, M., Gedo, J., Pollock, G., Sadow, L., & Sclessinger, N. (1969). Some aspects of Charcot's influence on Freud. In: *Freud: The Fusion of Science and Humanism*, ed. J. Gedo & G. Pollock. *Psychological Issues*, 34/35. New York: International Universities Press, 1976, pp. 115-132.

Montaigne, M. (1588). Of anger. In: *The Complete Essays*, trans. D. Frame. Stanford: Stanford University Press, 1958, pp. 539-545.

Murdoch, I. (1953). *Sartre: Romantic Rationalist*. New Haven: Yale University Press.

Ornstein, P., & Ornstein, A. (1985). Clinical understanding and explaining: The empathic vantage point. In: *Progress in Self Psychology*, Vol. 1, ed. A. Goldberg. New York: Guilford Press, pp. 43-61.

Oxford English Dictionary, Compact Edition. (1971). Oxford: Clarendon Press.

Papousek, H. (1975). Cognitive aspects of preverbal social interaction between human infants and adults. In: *Parent-Infant Interaction* (CIBA Foundation Symposium). New York: Associated Scientific Publishers.

Pollock, G. (1968). Josef Breuer. In: *Freud: The Fusion of Science and Humanism*, ed. J. Gedo, & G. Pollock, *Psychological Issues*, 34/35. New York: International Universities Press, 1976, pp. 133-163.

Richfield, J. (1954). An analysis of the concept of insight. *Psychoanalytic Quarterly*, 23:390-408.

Rycroft, C. (1968). *A Critical Dictionary of Psychoanalysis*. New York: Basic Books.

Sander, L. (1983). To begin with—Reflections on ontogeny. In: *Reflections on Self Psychology*, ed. J. Lichtenberg & S. Kaplan. Hillsdale, NJ: Analytic Press.

Sandler, J. (1976). Dreams, unconscious fantasies and "identity of perception." *International Review of Psychoanalysis*, 3:43-47.

Sartre, J.-P. (1938). *Nausea*. New York: New Directions, 1964.

Schwaber, E. (1979). On the "self" within the matrix of analytic theory—Some clinical reflections and considerations. *International Journal of Psychoanalysis*, 60:467-479.

——— (1984). Empathy: A mode of analytic listening. In: *Empathy II*, ed. J. Lichtenberg, M. Bornstein, & D. Silver. Hillsdale, NJ: Analytic Press, pp. 143-172.

Shane, M. (1985). Summary of Kohut's "The Self-Psychological Approach to Defense and Resistance." In: *Progress in Self Psychology*, Vol. 1, ed. A. Goldberg. New York: Guilford Press, pp. 69-79.

——— & Shane, E. (1984). The endphase of analysis: Indicators, functions, and task determination. *Journal of the American Psychoanalytic Association*, 32:739-772.

Stepansky, P., & Goldberg, A. (eds.). (1984). *Kohut's Legacy: Contributions to Self Psychology*. Hillsdale, NJ: Analytic Press.

Stern, D. (1974). Mother and infant at play: The dyadic interaction involving facial, vocal and gaze behavior. In: *The Effect of the Infant on its Caregiver*, ed. M. Lewis & L. Rosenbaum. New York: Wiley.

——— (1984). Affect attunement. In: *Frontiers of Infant Psychiatry*, Vol. 2, ed. J. D. Call, E. Galenson, & R. L. Tyson. New York: Basic Books.

——— (1985). *The Interpersonal world of the Infant*. New York: Basic Books.

Stolorow, R. D., & Lachmann, F. (1980). *Psychoanalysis of Developmental Arrests: Theory and Treatment*. New York: International Universities Press.

Stolorow, R., Brandchaft, B., & Atwood, G. (1987). *Psychoanalytic Treatment: An Intersubjective Approach*. Hillsdale, NJ: Analytic Press.

Strachey, J. (1934). The nature of the therapeutic action of psychoanalysis. Reprinted in: *International Journal of Psychoanalysis*, 1969, 50:275-292.

Strozier, C. (1985). Glimpses of a life: Heinz Kohut (1913-1981). In: *Progress in Self Psychology*, Vol. 1, ed. A. Goldberg. New York: Guilford Press, pp. 3-12.

Tolpin, M. (1971). On the beginnings of a cohesive self. In: *Psychoanalytic Study of the Child*, Vol. 26. New Haven: Yale University Press, pp. 273-305.

——— (1986). The self and its selfobjects: A different baby. In: *Progress in Self Psychology*, Vol. 2, ed. A. Goldberg. New York: Guilford Press, pp. 115-128.

Tolpin, P. (1980). The borderline personality: Its make-up and analyzability. In: *Advances in Self Psychology*, ed. A. Goldberg. New York: International Universities Press, pp. 299-316.

Weissman, S., & Cohen, R. (1985). The parenting alliance and adolescence. *Adolescent Psychiatry*, 12:24-45.

White, R. W. (1959). Motivation reconsidered: The concept of competence. In: *Psychological Review*, 66:292-333.

Winnicott, D. W. (1954). Metapsychological and clinical aspects of regression within the psychoanalytical set-up. In: *Collected Papers*. New York: Basic Books, 1958, pp. 278-294.

Wolf, E. S. (1976a). Ambience and abstinence. *Annual of Psychoanalysis*, 4:101-115.

——— (1976b). Recent advances in the psychology of the self: An outline of basic concepts. *Comprehensive Psychiatry*, 17:37-46.

——— (1978). The disconnected self: Modern sensibility in the writings of Kafka, Sartre and Virginia Woolf. In: *Psychoanalysis, Creativity and Literature*, ed. A. Roland. New York: Columbia University Press, pp. 103-114.

——— (1979). Transference and countertransference in the analysis of the disorders of the self. *Contemporary Psychoanalysis*, 15:577-594.

——— (1980a). The dutiful physician: The central role of empathy in psychoanalysis, psychotherapy and medical practice. *The Hillside Journal of Clinical Psychiatry*, 2:41-56.

——— (1980b). Introduction to "Self psychology and the concept of health." In: *Advances in Self Psychology*, ed. A. Goldberg. New York: International Universities Press, pp. 133-135.

——— (1980c). On the developmental line of selfobject relations. In: *Advances in Self Psychology*, ed. A. Goldberg. New York: International Universities Press, pp. 117-130.

——— (1980-1981). Psychoanalytic psychology of the self and literature. *New Literary History*, 12:41-60.

——— (1982). Comments on Heinz Kohut's conceptualization of a bipolar self. In: *Psychosocial Theories of the Self*, ed. B. Lee. New York: Plenum, pp. 23-42.

——— (1983). Empathy and Countertransference. In: *The Future of Psychoanalysis*, ed. A. Goldberg. New York: International Universities Press, pp. 309-326.

——— (1984a). Disruptions in the treatment of disorders of the self. In: *Kohut's*

Legacy, ed. P. Stepansky & A. Goldberg. Hillsdale, NJ: Analytic Press, pp. 143-156.

——— (1984b). The inevitability of interaction. *Psychoanalytic Inquiry*, 4:413-428.

——— (1985). The search for confirmation: Technical aspects of mirroring. *Psychoanalytic Inquiry*, 5:271-282.

——— Gedo, J., & Terman, D. (1972). On the adolescent process as a transformation of the self. *Journal of Youth and Adolescence*, 1:257-272.

——— & Wolf, I. P. (1979). We perished, each alone: A psychoanalytic commentary on Virginia Woolf's *To The Lighthouse*. *The International Review of Psychoanalysis*, 6:37-47.

APPENDIX I: MEDICATIONS

The following discussion of the use of psychopharmacological agents will deal with this complex and rapidly advancing field only from the point of view of the psychoanalyst. It is based on psychological principles and not on any special expertise in psychopharmacology. For the indications, pharmacology, and dosage of medications, the psychoanalytic therapist is well advised to work in collaboration with a qualified psychiatrist.

Therapists are quite divided in their opinions about the concomitant use of medications along with psychotherapy or psychoanalysis. Some believe very strongly that any use of medications for a strictly psychological illness is contra-indicated because it interferes, they think, with the proper unfolding of the therapeutic process. Furthermore, there is also the possibility of distorting the transference relationship to the therapist who prescribes medications, because he will be seen as acting, to some extent, in a magical and parental fashion that distracts from his role as the mere co-interpreter of the psychodynamic processes he observes.

On the other hand, many, perhaps the majority of psychotherapists, seem to believe that these threats to the psychotherapeutic process arising from the concomitant prescription of medications are more theoretical than real. It is my impression that the giving of medications to patients in psychotherapeutic treatment is quite common and felt to be helpful by many patients as well as therapists.

In my psychoanalytic as well as in my psychotherapeutic practice I attempt to tailor my approach to the individual patient. As a general guideline I would prefer the use of psychological methods over pharmacological ones. However, there are occasions when the use of psychopharmacological agents can support and enhance the psychological efforts. For example, some depressed patients are unable to make the efforts required by psychotherapeutic work unless their symptoms are somewhat relieved by antidepressant medications. Similarly, some chronically anxious patients will do better in treatment when the therapy is supplemented by anxiolytic drugs. This is particularly true for that variety of patients with phobic symptomatology. However, in view of the rapid advances being made, I find it impossible to remain sufficiently up-to-date in both psychoanalytic and psychopharmacologic practice. In general, therefore, when the use of medication appears indicated, whether in addition to or instead of psychotherapeutic endeavors, I work in consultative collaboration with a colleague specializing in psychopharmacologic management or refer the patient to him.

Many patients attach idiosyncratic meanings to the agents they are taking. Some patients experience the medications as a token of the special care and concern of the therapist. Others view any active pharmacological agent very suspiciously as a potential intruder into their mind and feel threatened in the integrity of their self. They would rather suffer pain and discomfort than worry about whether their thought processes are still their own. Though such troubling thoughts may seem quite irrational and far removed from reality to the therapist, the patient's experience should be respected. No pressure should be brought to bear on the patient to take medication against his or her wishes unless considerations of safety, for example, suicidal or homicidal possibilities, or other dangerous acting out, make a forceful intervention necessary. In such cases the therapist must be aware that his actions may precipitate a paranoid development and may make any future psychotherapeutic collaboration impossible.

APPENDIX II:
THIRD-PARTY RELATIONS

Psychoanalytic treatment initiates a process that gradually involves increasingly deeper layers of the personality. Inevitably, the most intimate and private thoughts, feelings, and fantasies of the patient—but also, to a more limited extent, of the therapist—become the very materials that fuel the analytic and therapeutic processes. The potential exposure of one's innermost life to the possible disdain of someone else or even to the condemnation by one's self is greatly feared. We have seen in earlier chapters how this arouses resistance and how much painstaking effort goes into creating the ambience and making the proper interpretation to overcome the resistance when the therapeutic situation is open to only the two participating individuals. The presence of third parties would increase the obstacles to the evolution of a therapeutic process immeasurably and is generally avoided in adult therapy whenever possible.

Yet third-party interference in psychotherapeutic and psychoanalytic work is as common as it is annoying to both therapist and patient. The ill effects of such interference when they prevent the necessary frequency of sessions or when they halt them altogether are obvious. Many patients can be treated successfully with psychoanalytic methods when circumstances allow a sufficient frequency of sessions to facilitate the requisite intensity of the mobilized affects. The patient can allow himself the required painful self-exploration only when he has the assurance of being able to discuss newly emerging memories and their associated feelings almost immediately with the empathic and understanding therapist. Even psychologically sophisticated individuals who are well disposed to depth-psychological treatment often find it difficult to understand that increasing sessions from, let us say, twice a week to four or five times a week, often makes the difference between success and failure of the therapeutic endeavor. This does not mean, however, that every patient should be in analysis, nor that every analytic patient need be seen rigidly four or five times a week. In my experience one can do good analytic work with some people in three-times-a-week sessions. Increasing the frequency, continuity, and intensity of the work, however, would have enhanced its effectiveness.

Insurance companies increasingly ask for fairly detailed information about a patient's diagnosis and treatment. This intrusion threatens the confidentiality of the doctor–patient relationship and therefore becomes a threat to the therapeutic process itself. The success of any psychotherapeutic effort worth its name depends on the ability of the patient to reveal his innermost thoughts and feelings to the therapist without having to fear that these will be revealed to others. The whole therapeutic enterprise is in jeopardy when confidentiality cannot be maintained. However, so far, in my experience, it has been possible for me to fill out questionnaires with responses that are adequate to the insurer's needs without seriously breaching confidentiality. But the pressure on therapists to break confidentiality appears likely to increase and calls for vigilance and resistance.

Pressure to break confidentiality can also come from parents, spouses, friends, and employers. Usually, these are well-meaning people who don't realize how destructive it would be to the therapeutic process if the therapist complied. Not only is it detrimental to break confidentiality, but many patients would be disturbed by almost any communication between their therapists and others about themselves. For the sake of keeping a therapeutic process going, or of allowing one to get established at all, it is necessary that therapists keep contacts with adult patients' friends and family to an absolute, unavoidable minimum.

GLOSSARY OF
SELF PSYCHOLOGY TERMS

Competitive Aggressiveness is a form of potentially violent aggression that aims to forcefully overcome an obstacle which is blocking a goal satisfaction of a self. Competitive aggressiveness disappears spontaneously when the frustration has been overcome.

Efficacy Need is a person's need to experience the self as an effective agent, that is, capable of eliciting a selfobject response. The associated *efficacy pleasure* appears to be derived from the enhanced awareness of the self having been strengthened through the experience of efficacy.

Empathy, according to Kohut, is synonymous with vicarious introspection. It is a process of gaining access to another's psychological state by feeling oneself into the other's experience (cf. Freud's [1913a] use of *Einfuehlung*). The reliability of empathy in obtaining psychoanalytic data depends on training and experience in its controlled use, as well as on careful self-monitoring of potential countertransferential distortions. Empathy is not to be confused with sympathy or kindness, nor does it designate an affective attitude. It is simply a method of data collection.

Narcissistic Rage is a form of potentially violent aggression that aims to destroy an offending selfobject when this selfobject is experienced as threatening the continued cohesion or existence of the self, particularly when this threat to the self takes the form of imposing helplessness on the self. Narcissistic rage does not disappear when the threat to the self disappears; rather, it lingers smolderingly in readiness to burst again into violent rage at the slightest real or perceived provocation. It will fade gradually, however, when another selfobject's empathic understanding can be trusted and accepted.

Narcissistic Transference. See Selfobject Transference.

Self, according to Kohut, is a depth-psychological concept that refers to the core of the personality, which is made up of various constituents that emerge into a coherent and enduring configuration during the interplay of inherited and environmental factors with the child's experience of its earliest selfobjects. Each self has a history, that is, a past, a present, and a future. As a unit that endures over time, it develops in the lawful gradual manner of a psychological structure. Among its core attributes, the self is the center of initiative, recipient of impressions, and repository of that individual's particular constellation of nuclear ambitions, ideals, talents, and skills. These motivate and permit it to function as a self-propelling, self-directed, and self-sustaining unit, which provides a central purpose to the personality and gives a sense of meaning to the person's life. The patterns of ambitions, skills, and goals, the tensions between them, the program of action they create, and the resultant activities that shape the individual's life are all experienced as continuous in space and time and give the person a sense of selfhood as an independent center of initiative and independent center of impressions.

Constituents of the self are (1) a pole from which emanate the basic strivings for power and recognition, (2) a pole that maintains the guiding ideals, and (3) an arc of tension between the two poles that activates the basic talents and skills. Kohut initially termed the self that he described the *bipolar self* to emphasize the bipolar structure, that is, the pole of ambitions and the pole of ideals, and to distinguish it from other descriptions of the self in the literature.

Since the self is found to have characteristic attributes depending on the level of its development and on its structural state, self psychology has described various *types* of self concepts or self states:

• the *virtual* self is the image of the neonate's self as it resides in the parent's mind and thus determines how the parents address the neonate's as yet unformed self potentials. In so doing, they shape these potentials so that when this self first emerges as a cohesive structure sometime during the second year of life, it is termed the *nuclear* self.

• the *cohesive* self describes the relatively coherent structure of the normally and healthily functioning self.

• the *grandiose* self describes the early infantile exhibitionistic self that blissfully experiences itself normally as the omnipotent center of all existence.

• the *fragmented* self describes the lessened coherency of the self resulting from faulty selfobject responses or from other regression-producing conditions. Depending on the degree of fragmentation, it can be experienced along a continuum from mildly anxious disconcertedness to the panic of total loss of self structure.

• the *empty* self describes the loss of vigor and depression consequent upon depletion of the self's energies resulting from lack of joyful responses to its existence and assertiveness.

• the *overburdened* self is deficient in self-soothing capacity because it has not been provided with the opportunity to merge with the calmness of an omnipotent selfobject.

• the *overstimulated* self is prone to recurrent states of excessive emotionality or excitement as the result of unempathically excessive or phase-inappropriate responses from the selfobjects of childhood.

• the *imbalanced* self maintains its precarious cohesion by overemphasis on one of the major constituents at the expense of the other two. One variety is psychopathically ambitious without the proper guidance from the pole of values, because the latter is relatively weak *vis-à-vis* the pole of ambitions. Another variety is guilt-ridden and overly constrained from an excessively strong pole of values. A third variety is characterized by relatively weak poles with an excessive emphasis on the tension arc between the poles, along which the inborn talents and learned skills are arrayed. Consequently, this imbalance produces, for example, the technical specialist who is dedicated to the perfection of competence without the normal regard for issues of personal ambition or ethical values. Gradations may vary from the quasi-normal "organization man" to the near-psychotic Adolf Eichmann.

Self Psychology is an elaboration and development by Heinz Kohut and his colleagues of the psychoanalytic concepts of narcissism and the self. Self psychology is characterized by emphasis on the vicissitudes of the structure of the self and of the associated subjective conscious and unconscious experience of selfhood. Self psychology recognizes as the most fundamental essence of human psychology the individual's need (1) to organize his or her psychological experience into a cohesive configuration, the self, and (2) to establish self-sustaining relationships between this self and its surround that have the function to evoke, maintain, and strengthen the structural coherence, energic vigor, and balanced harmony among the constituents of the self.

The field of study of self psychology is co-extensive with that of psychoanalysis generally, that is, depthpsychology. The methodology of this field is defined by the use of vicarious introspection, that is, empathy (see definition), as a necessary participant, in conjunction with other observations, in the process of data collection. Insistence on rigorous adherence to scientific standards of data evaluation, together with conceptual clarity of theories and hypotheses as well as noncontradictory contiguity with other related sciences of man, are tenets designed to insure scientific soundness, respectability, and acceptance.

Selfobject is a term often used imprecisely to describe the form, or the function, or the participating persons or objects in the specific types of relationships that are associated with the structuring of the self. Precisely defined, a selfobject is neither self nor object, but the *subjective* aspect of a self-sustaining function performed by a relationship of self to objects who by their presence or activity evoke and maintain the self and the experience of selfhood. As such, the selfobject relationship refers to an intrapsychic experience and does not describe the interpersonal relationship between the self and other objects. It denotes the experience of imagoes that are needed for the sustenance of the self.

The relationship to specific *types* of selfobjects can be described by reference to their specific functions:

* *infantile* selfobjects normally sustain the self of early infancy. When the need for these is chronic or revived during adulthood, they are spoken of as *archaic* selfobjects, thus implying some degree of pathology.

* *mirroring* selfobjects sustain the self by providing the experience of acceptance and confirmation of the self in its grandness, goodness, and wholeness.

* *idealizable* selfobjects sustain the self by allowing it the experience of merger with the calmness, power, wisdom, and goodness of the idealized selfobject.

• *alter-ego* selfobjects sustain the self by providing the experience of a perceptible presence of essential likeness of another's self.

• *adversarial* selfobjects sustain the self by providing the experience of being a center of initiative through permitting nondestructive oppositional self-assertiveness.

Selfobject Disorders (also called Self Disorders), as designated by Kohut, are characterized by significant failure of the self to achieve cohesion, vigor, or harmony, or by a significant loss of these qualities after they had become tentatively established. Major clinical diagnostic categories always imply damage to the self's structural integrity and strength, secondary to faulty selfobject responsiveness. Consequently, the cohesion, vigor, or harmony of these structures is impaired and the resulting conditions can be described as follows:

• *Psychosis* is that selfobject disorder where serious damage to the self is either permanent or protracted and when no defensive structures cover the defect. An inherent biological tendency is generally assumed to be a necessary antecedent in conjunction with the psychological etiological factors damaging the self.

• *Borderline States* are those selfobject disorders where serious damage to the self is either permanent or protracted, but where the experiential and behavioral manifestations of the defect are covered by complex defenses.

• *Narcissistic Behavior Disorders* are those selfobject disorders where the damage to the self is temporary and restorable through appropriate psychoanalytic treatment and where the symptoms express an alloplastic attempt to force the environment to yield needed selfobject experiences via behavioral maneuvers (*e.g.*, soothing responses in interpersonal relationships) or to yield perceptions of restored selfobject functioning (*e.g.*, addiction, perversion, delinquency).

• *Narcissistic Personality Disorders* are those selfobject disorders where the damage to the self is temporary and restorable through appropriate psychoanalytic treatment and where the symptoms express the tensions associated with damage to the self or the tensions of autoplastic attempts to restore selfobject functioning (*e.g.*, hypochondria, depression, hypersensitivity, lack of zest).

• *Depressions* were divided by Kohut into 3 types. *Preverbal*: apathy, sense of deadness, and diffuse rage related to primordial trauma. *Empty*: depletion of self-esteem and vitality consequent upon lack of joyful selfobject responses, leading the self to experience itself in a world of unmirrored ambitions or in a world devoid of ideals. *Guilt*: depression characterized by the spreading of unrealistically heightened self-rejection and self-blame consequent on deprivation of the repeated experience of participating in the calmness of an idealized adult—that is, of merger with an idealized selfobject—during crucial periods of self-formation.

Selfobject Transference is the displacement on to the analyst of the analysand's needs for a responsive selfobject matrix, derived in part from remobilized and regressively altered editions of archaic infantile selfobject needs, in part from current age- and phase-appropriate selfobject needs, and in part from selfobject needs mobilized in response to the analyst and the analytic situation. Selfobject transferences manifest through the expression of direct or of implied demands on the analyst or through defenses against the expression of these demands. Specific types are described as follows:

• *Merger transference* is the re-establishment of an identity with the (self)object of early development through an extension of the self to include the analyst in it. It manifests by an expectation that the analyst not be a center of initiative, but that he be subject to the patient's initiative, for example, like the patient's limbs. Sometimes the expectation includes that the analyst be so attuned to the patient's needs and thoughts that he know them without explicitly being told by the patient.

• *Mirror transference* was used by Kohut as a generic term that included merger transference, alter-ego transference, and mirror transference proper in contradistinction to the idealizing transference. Among these mirror transferences, the mirror transference proper referred to the re-establishment of an early need for acceptance and confirmation of the self by the selfobject matrix. The mirror transference proper manifests as demands on the analyst (or defenses against such demands) to recognize, admire, or praise the patient. See also under selfobject transference, merger transference, alter-ego transference, idealizing transference.

• *Alter-ego transference* is the re-establishment of a latency need to see and understand, as well as to be seen and be understood by someone like oneself. Kohut initially classified the alter-ego transference as one of the generic type of mirror transferences, but later emphasized it as a separate type of transference. It manifests as a need, in general, to be like the analyst in appearance, manner, outlook, and opinion. Developmentally, the alter-ego relationship is associated with the fantasy of an imaginary playmate and may also be important in the acquisition of skills and competences.

• *Idealizing transference* is the re-establishment of the need for merging with a calm, strong, wise, and good selfobject. It may manifest as the more or less disguised admiration of the analyst, his character and values, or by defenses against this transference, such as prolonged and bitter depreciation of the analyst.

• *Transference of creativity* is Kohut's term for the transient need of certain creative personalities for merger with a selfobject while engaged in the most taxing creative tasks. An example might be Freud's need for Fliess during the writing of *The Interpretation of Dreams* (1900).

Splitting: The self may split either horizontally or vertically, according to Kohut. In the *horizontal split*, painful fantasies and other unacceptable ideational material originating from within the psyche are kept out of consciousness. For example, a grandiose fantasy about the self may be kept repressed via the horizontal split to protect against painful exposure to reality, and such an individual may experience himself, therefore, as chronically inferior, weak, and depressed. In the *vertical split*, percepts of external reality are disavowed or denied. Thus, for example, an individual may consciously know that a loved one has died, but due to a vertical split disavow this knowledge and thus be protected from the painful impact of such a loss, with the result that affectively he will act as if this death had not occurred.

Transmuting Internalization is Kohut's term for a process of structure formation in which aspects of the function of the self–selfobject transaction are internalized under the pressure generated by optimal frustration.

INDEX